# VIGOR REGAINED

## A Simple, Proven Home Program for Restoring Fitness and Vitality

# VIGOR REGAINED

## A Simple, Proven Home Program for Restoring Fitness and Vitality

by

Dr. Herbert A. deVries



PRENTICE-HALL, INC.
Englewood Cliffs, New Jersey

*VIGOR REGAINED: A Simple, Proven Home Program for Restoring Fitness and Vitality*
by Dr. Herbert A. deVries



Printed in the United States of America

Prentice-Hall International, Inc., London
Prentice-Hall of Australia, Pty. Ltd., North Sidney
Prentice-Hall of Canada, Ltd., Toronto
Prentice-Hall of India Private Ltd., New Delhi
Prentice-Hall of Japan, Inc., Tokyo

10 9 8 7 6 5 4 3 2

---

Library of Congress Cataloging in Publication Data

deVries, Herbert A. Vigor regained.

Includes bibliographical references.
1. Aged--Care and hygiene. 2. Exercise--Physiological effect. I. Title.
[DNLM: 1. Gymnastics--In old age.
2. Physical fitness--Popular works.
QT225 D514v 1974]
RC952.D413 613.7'1'0240565
73-17384 ISBN 0-13-942169-6

*To my favorite jogging partner and typist
who just happens also to be my wife, Lorane deVries,
who serves breakfast pre-dawn in order to join
me on the beach at dawn. Her health benefits
from the active life have exceeded my own.*

# Preface

Ideally, physical fitness is a condition which should be achieved in youth, pursued in middle age, and never relinquished. Yet, as we have documented in our studies, it can also be developed in the later years by persons who have led previously sedentary lives. This book shows how men and women can attain fitness safely and effectively.

The book is written in response to a real need among older generations of our society. Few persons who grew up and attended school in the early decades of this century were fortunate enough to have the excellent physical education programs offered in so many of our schools today. Gymnasiums and swimming pools were still among the luxuries coveted by all school districts but possessed by very few. Physiologists had not yet shown very great interest in the health benefits to be had from physical fitness. Further, these same generations are now mature citizens of the technological age, in which hard physical work is largely a thing of the past and exercise is done too little if at all.

In view of the lack of physical conditioning experienced by older generations, and the advances of modern medicine, it is not surprising that disease statistics have shown marked changes in the last forty years or so. Infectious diseases such as poliomyelitis, tuberculosis, and smallpox have been virtually eradicated. They have been replaced, however, by coronary heart disease, arteriosclerosis, diabetes, arthritis, and other diseases of the degenerative type. Laboratory research has shown that degeneration can be caused by disuse. Indeed, one is prompted to believe that our legacy of degenerative disease may be related at least in part to our newly-found lifestyle of lazy leisure living.

The fact that use improves function and disuse results in dysfunction is known to every physiologist. But this information has not been impressed sufficiently on the lay public. In fact, much of what has passed for knowledge in the area of physical fitness and health maintenance has been produced by faddists and cultists. Again, the need for a book such as this, based on scientific fact, is obvious.

This book also is a response to substantial public demand. After the publicity generated by our laboratory work with older men and women, I was besieged with personal letters from older persons requesting instructions on how to exercise to achieve the health benefits our research was beginning to suggest. In answer to those who wrote and to thousands of others interested in improving their health, this book provides the only program of its kind for older people, with a unique self-testing and self-monitoring component to ensure safety and effectiveness.

I would like to express my gratitude to the older men and women of Laguna Hills, California, Leisure World retirement community, who helped make this book possible. As willing and enthusiastic research subjects, they enabled me to establish that physical fitness is for all ages and can be successfully pursued in the later years as well as in youth.

I owe a special debt of gratitude to Mr. Michael Briley for his extensive assistance in preparing my material for publication. He is responsible for changing my writing style into language more easily understood by laymen, for whom this book is written.

Among the many others whose assistance made this book

possible were those associated with our laboratory research program sponsored by the Administration on Aging (U.S. Department of Health, Education and Welfare). I wish to thank Mr. Gene Adams, who was my research assistant in the laboratory and who gradually took over from me the leadership of the exercise program, and Mrs. Irene Lamberts, our only laboratory technician for some period of time.

After we reach fifty years of age, our need for physical fitness is probably even more critical than in our younger years. One of my greatest inspirations has been the sight of healthy men and women in their seventies and eighties achieving levels of vigor that are not ordinarily associated even with those thirty years younger. It is my fond hope that this book will stimulate you to do as much for yourself.

Herbert A. deVries

# Contents

# VIGOR REGAINED

## A Simple, Proven Home Program for Restoring Fitness and Vitality

# 1

# AND PROMISES TO KEEP . . .

## Our Research Program

At age 87, W. K., retired minister and educator, was as active as he could be.

Despite physical limitations from the discomforts and fatigue associated with advanced age, W. K. had much to accomplish in advancement of humanitarian causes. In the words of Robert Frost, he had "miles to go and promises to keep."

He was intrigued by our notice in the newspaper serving the Laguna Hills, California, Leisure World retirement community. It announced that an experimental exercise program for elderly persons was seeking volunteer participants. The program's aim, the article said, was to determine scientifically whether carefully planned and controlled exercise can help restore vigor to older people.

Because the prerequisite to participating in the program was a complete physical examination, W. K. consulted his physician. "You're too old," was the doctor's first reaction to the idea. But a thorough going-over revealed no symptom or impediment which would preclude a carefully controlled regimen of exercise. The doctor recommended him to us as a program participant.

A few days later, W. K. reported among our first class of exercisers as the senior member in a group of mere "youngsters" in their sixties and seventies. Because of his advanced age, we monitored him carefully through a specially designed, somewhat less strenuous routine than we conducted with the younger subjects. We urged him to go at his own pace in a modified walk/jog regimen, not competing with anyone. He was an active participant in these and other exercises for 18 months.

W. K. and the majority of the other persons who participated in our programs were very enthusiastic. We are most grateful to them. Their interest and cooperation transcended that motivated purely by personal gain. Importantly, they were an integral and necessary part of our research.

There is no longer any doubt that exercise is a must for the health of young people. It also is being confirmed that a vigorously active life benefits those in middle age. But what of the older person? Can you take a person past 50 who has rarely exercised strenuously and expect to improve his or her health with an exercise program? In short, the question is whether a person past 50 who has been bogged down in a sedentary life is also beyond the age when exercise can be introduced safely and effectively?

### Is the Program Really Beneficial to Older People?

Many have believed that exercise can be beneficial to older people, but there has been little scientific proof of this assumption. Some authorities, on the other hand, have claimed that a person who has been relatively inactive throughout his life cannot benefit from exercise in advancing age. But my experience of many years studying the effects of exercise made me unwilling to accept such a conclusion. It has been demonstrated that persons of any age, even the young, lose their vigor if they are deprived of physical activity. Several years ago, I was associated with a University of Southern California aerospace medicine study, dubbed "Operation Sacktime." This study showed that when a group of young healthy college men were kept in bed and inactive for two to three weeks, they lost (temporarily) the ability to adjust to strenuous activity, in functions of the heart, lungs, circulation, and muscles. In other words, they lost what we call vigor.

Coupling these observations with the realization that the majority of us no longer live an active life in our mature years, I questioned even further: If both aging and inactivity bring about the same basic effect—loss of vigor—how can we be certain that loss of vigor in older persons is due entirely to the processes of aging? Isn't it logical to think that some part of the physical decline we see in older people is the result of an inactive life? And, therefore, might it not be possible to reverse at least part of this decline?

It was this sort of logic that prompted me to propose to the Administration of Aging of the U.S. Department of Health, Education and Welfare, that the agency underwrite us in a scientific study. Happily the AOA saw fit to support us for two years in the endeavor. Working under the auspices of the University of Southern California's Ethel Percy Andrus Gerontology Center, we set up a mobile research facility at Laguna Hills Leisure World in order to take the laboratory to the people.

**Good News**

Preliminary results of the program were not long in coming. "Good News for Joggers" boomed the headline in *Time* magazine:

> *Joggers—like religious fanatics—must be endowed with an abundance of faith. They assume that physical exercise is good for them, but there has been relatively little scientific evidence to back them up. Now Herbert A. deVries, a University of Southern California physical education professor, has conducted before-and-after tests and has found, he contends, that exercise makes the bodies of septuagenarians act like those of 40-year-olds.*
>
> *Gathering 41 far-from-athletic oldsters ranging in age from 50 to 87, deVries gave them complete physical examinations, tested reactions, then put them through hour-long workouts three times a week. Puffing at first, the late-blooming physical culturists engaged in calisthenics, jogging, stretching and water exercises. Within six weeks the difference between the exercisers and a nonexercising group of 26 men in the same age range was profound.*
>
> *Repetitions of the tests showed that deVries' subjects averaged a 4.9% drop in body fat, a 6% reduction in diastolic blood pressure, a 9.2% rise in maximum oxygen*

*consumption (the best single index of vigor, according to deVries), and a 7.2% increase in the strength of their arms. Perhaps more important, if more debatable, was deVries' conclusion from measuring the electrical activity of muscles. He equates these pulses with nervous tension and says that his exercisers cut tension by 15%. . . .*[1]

The "Good News" bannered by *Time* was exactly that for 87-year-old W. K. After just a month and a half of exercising one hour three times a week, dramatic improvements in certain measures of his physical function began to appear. He could perform at increasing workloads for a longer time. His heart and lungs were transporting life-sustaining oxygen throughout his system more efficiently and with less effort. His maximal oxygen consumption, the best single measure of an individual's vigor, had increased significantly. After a year and a half in the program, his blood pressure had dropped markedly toward

**Figure 1-1 AOA group exercising. (Allan D. Walker)**

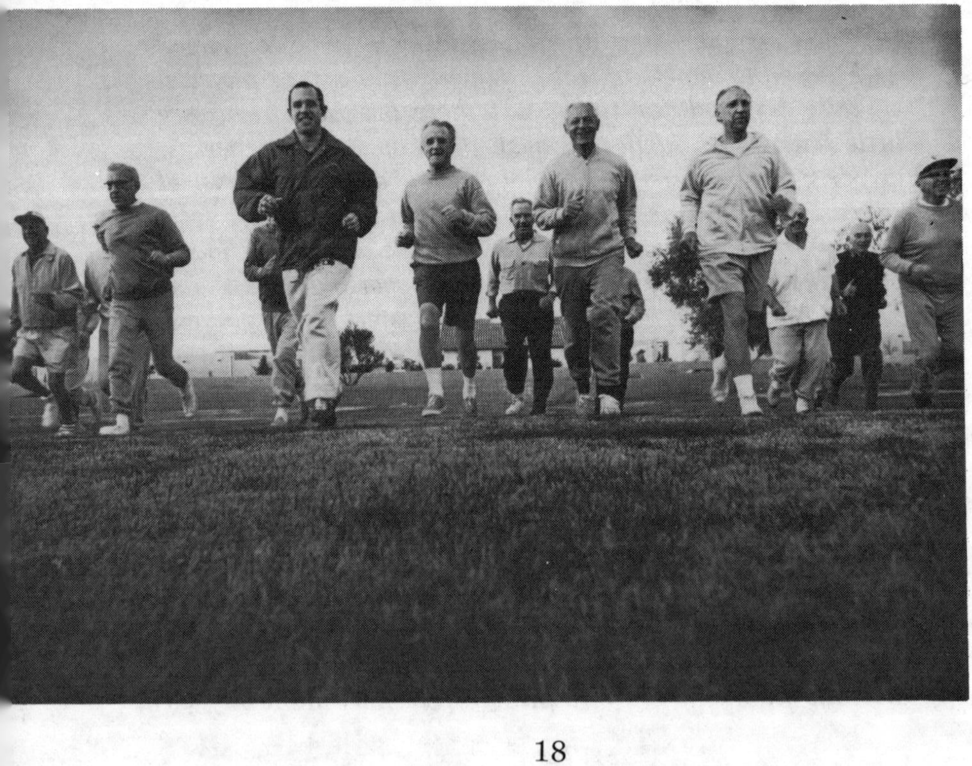

normal ranges. He already had experienced a gradual but pronounced trend in his ability to relax. Never having been athletic in his younger years, he was particularly enthusiastic that the first strenuous exercise on a regular basis in his life had restored some of his lost vigor.

**You, Too, Can Feel Much Younger**

Now bright-eyed and sprightly in his early nineties, W. K. continues with exercise, walking several miles per week at a fast clip. Exercise, he says, "has made a much younger man of me." It requires less effort now for him to be active in public speaking and promotion of scholarships for needy students. Tiring less readily, he finds walking and other physical efforts much easier than before. Prior to starting the exercise program, he had a lifetime history of headaches about twice a week, relieved only by taking large doses of aspirin. After he began the program, he says, the need for aspirin gradually was reduced. After 14 months of exercise three times a week, he no longer needed any aspirin. He previously had been conscious of constant discomfort in his lower back, sometimes to the point of pain. Now, he says, "I no longer know I have a back."

The *Time* article was accurate in reporting early results of our study. The differences due to exercise in the 41 "far-from-athletic oldsters" were indeed profound. It is true that in terms of physical function, some persons in their seventies did regain the vigor of their forties. Although their chronological age might have been 70-plus, their "physiological age" had been reduced 20 to 30 years in terms of accepted norms for oxygen consumption and transport, blood pressure, and other indicators. The majority of our subjects registered substantial improvements; every one benefited to some extent.

And the "Good News" was even better by the end of the study. Its continuation eventually involved more than 100 subjects, all of whom were tested at six weeks, and some of whom were followed for 42 weeks. The six weeks' results reported by *Time* were confirmed, and in many cases were shown to be conservative.[2] Although the most dramatic changes appeared in about six weeks, the improvements on a group average continued in an upward trend, at a slower rate, between the 18-week and 42-week intervals, and in some cases beyond. Therefore, we had realized one of the major goals of our research study: We had concluded that carefully planned and controlled exercise can be both safe and beneficial for older people. We had proven finally the inaccuracy of theories that persons who led sedentary lives in their younger years cannot be improved by exercise in their mature years. On the contrary, we found that the ones who had been least active in youth and middle age benefited the most from the exercise program.

### Other People Who Have Benefited from the Program

Another of our subjects was a 68-year-old retiree who in his work had been accustomed to a good deal of physical effort, including stooping, lifting, and bending. Although he had been relatively active throughout his life, he has come to believe that to get the most out of physical activity "you have to work your arms and legs and get your heart going" in a regular program as the groups did in our prescribed jogging, swimming, calisthenics, and stretching exercises. His contention seems to be borne out in the program's results for him: He reports that after just two months in the program, he eliminated the need for cathartics and laxatives. He also says troublesome kinks in the back and tendonitis and bursitis around his knee joints disappeared in that length of time. He was always a fairly good sleeper, but he sleeps even better now. He says he has doubled his frequency of sexual intercourse.

One man who started the program at 70 had suffered from mild emphysema since age 55. He is now able to run as far as one-and-a-quarter miles without stopping and has much less difficulty in breathing than before beginning the exercise program. He reports a "feeling of accomplishment and general well-being."

Many more of the older people who participated in this and other of our studies have told us of improvements in how they feel as the result of our controlled exercise program. More endurance, fewer aches and pains, and increased relaxation are recurring themes in their conversations with us. Some of our male subjects' wives have commented, too: Their husbands are easier to live with since they have been exercising, the women say.

### Request for More Information from All Over the World

In early 1969, following the *Time* article, an Associated Press account, and other stories about our work which appeared in newspapers across the nation and the world, we were deluged by letters. In addition to several hundred which came from throughout the U.S., we received letters from such distant points as Taiwan, Brazil, Pakistan, Mozambique, Canada, Australia, Germany, England, Argentina, Japan, and Mexico. The writers represented a wide range of professions concerned with the well-being of older people. Included were recreation specialists, physicians, university researchers, physical therapists, coaches, social workers, senior citizens' program administrators, nurses, graduate students, and YMCA officials. All were interested in obtaining further information about our studies of exercise for the elderly. But probably the majority of the letters came from older individuals wanting to learn how to proceed with exercise that would benefit them as it did the men who participated in our program.

It is to them, and to millions of other healthy older men and women who have potential for a more vigorous life, that this book is dedicated and addressed. Designed to eliminate guesswork, it is an accurate account of our research findings. Based on firm scientific evidence, it will relate the benefits of exercise in terms of basic, physical functions as we have documented them, using our own techniques and instrumentation. Our prescription for exercise, contained in later pages, is designed to tell the reader how to go about it in a safe and effective manner.

To put the results of our work into correct perspective: We are not saying that exercise promises to cure headaches, restore regularity, enliven the sex life, and do away with aches and pains. Neither we nor anyone else has scientific data to substantiate such a claim. Nonetheless, these very real effects have been reported by some of our research subjects. We can say only that it seems reasonable to believe that the disappearance of headaches, for example, may well be related to the decrease in nervous tension and the lowering of blood pressure which are brought about by planned exercise. We have scientifically demonstrated significant improvements in basic function through such exercise. These improvements may be manifested in many positive side effects.

Another point I wish to clarify, at the outset, is that we have not discovered the fabled Fountain of Youth, nor was it our intent to do so. There is no evidence to suggest that better physical fitness will lengthen the lifespan. Nevertheless, we maintain that the headline in *Time*, "Good News for Joggers," is an accurate appraisal.

We reaffirm that virtually every normal, healthy older person can rejuvenate himself to some degree through carefully planned and controlled exercise. Exercise might not add years to your life, but it does hold the rich promise of adding life to your years.

# 2

# THE MATURE GENERATION . . .

## Exercise For You

Welcome to the "Nation of the Retired."

The phrase is no exaggeration. It describes a "nation" emerging within our own country. There are now more than 28.5 million Americans over 60—more than the entire populations of Sweden, Norway, Denmark, Finland, and Switzerland combined. Even the number of Americans over 65 is approaching that of the entire population of Canada. Estimates say there will be about 25 million U.S. citizens over 65 by the year 2000.

Dr. James E. Birren, director of the University of Southern California's Ethel Percy Andrus Gerontology Center, coined the phrase, "Nation of the Retired." Birren contends that it not only describes a growing group within a country but also has something to say about our nation as a whole. "The U.S. has a youth-oriented culture and an image as a young country, but in terms of the growing proportion of older population, we are becoming an 'old' nation," Birren says.

As the birthrate falls in the U.S., the proportion of older persons in the population is rising. In the last century, 30 years have been added to the life expectancy of the average person in this country, and an increasing number of individuals has survived to reach old age. Also, with union contracts providing for retirement after 30 years of work, many persons will be retired at 55 or earlier and will spend 45 years outside the labor force as compared to only 30 in it.

The statistics tell the story: Those approaching mature age at present do so under a combination of life circumstances unique in history. Leonard Davis, honorary president of the American Association of Retired Persons and the National Retired Teachers Association, summed up this uniqueness concisely in a 1970 speech at the University of Southern California. He pointed out that the current retirement generation is facing "problems and challenges that no generation has been required or allowed to face before."

> *Until this era, man's lifespan had proceeded according to a predictable plan. The poets might write of the "seven ages of man," but, practically speaking, there were only* two. *The time until a person began to work—and the rest of his life during which he worked. Life expectancy was increasing rapidly, but the pattern was merely extended, not changed.*
>
> *And then, abruptly, it was changed. At age 65 the life cycle as it had been known for centuries was to terminate. But beyond that, a new segment, a new phase of life was to begin. There were no precedents for how to live this new segment. There were not even to be familiar responsibilities and routines on which to build. In other words, at the peak of maturity, people were to receive an almost stunning gift of life itself—as much as 25 years, or one-third of the Biblical lifespan—in which to live and find meaning in whatever way they chose and as long as they were permitted to remain physically and mentally able. . . .*

You're over 50, and what does this mean to you? One aspect is that you're a pioneer, in a sense, as a member of a new sort of "population explosion" of your age group. Retired or not, you're part of a very important segment of society. By sheer dint of numbers, alone, it has become a force to be reckoned with. No longer can our culture orient itself solely to the young, to the exclusion of the older population. Youth must be served, but so too must the mature generation.

However, despite the need for much to be accomplished, the picture for today's senior citizen is not a bleak one. The very fact that the sciences combined in the relatively new super-discipline of gerontology are growing in achievement and personnel so rapidly is a favorable indication. Across the land, there appears to be a stirring—an awakening of attention to the issues connected with our older population. The government, professions, churches, social agencies, educational institutions, and private enterprise (to a lesser extent) are beginning to heed the call. Organizations such as the American Association of Retired Persons and the National Retired Teachers Association, with their numerous programs and services, are indeed helping older Americans to achieve retirement lives of independence, dignity, and purpose. Significantly, members of the two organizations, in hundreds of thousands of individual donations, contributed more than half the construction cost of USC's Ethel Percy Andrus Gerontology Center, named in honor of the late founder of AARP and NRTA.

A refreshing view of old age was voiced by the psychologist, A. E. David Schonfield, in a news interview some years ago when he was a visiting professor at USC. Contending that "the Geritol Set is better off in many ways than the Pepsi Generation," Schonfield listed advantages of growing older which he found in a research study involving senior citizens.

"The overall picture we obtained is of an older group with fewer negative emotions than the young. The senior citizens we questioned showed a realistic perspective and enjoy social relations, revelling in the fact that they are not at the beck and call of society. They said the greatest advantages of old age are a lessening of the burdens of responsibility and time to do things—travel, read, visit the theater and nurture friendships."[1] Schonfield cautioned, of course, against getting too rosy a picture of old age, noting that the persons interviewed were reasonably healthy and relatively financially secure. It's right to assume that older persons who are financially deprived or beset with poor health would be burdened with worry and anxiety, just as persons of any age in the same circumstances would be. But he stressed that aging in itself does not mean the end of meaningful life—far from it.

Harking back to Leonard Davis's remarks, you have "an almost stunning gift of life . . . one-third of the Biblical life-span . . . in which to live and find meaning." But take note of the qualifier: As long as you "remain physically and mentally able." Prolonging the healthy and productive middle years is the thrust of gerontology. This is a compelling and exciting challenge. For me, having had the opportunity to make some small contribution in helping older persons improve their physical capacity for living has been one of the most rewarding experiences of my career. Nothing has been more inspiring to me than seeing our well-conditioned participants working and playing with renewed vigor.

### A New Sense of Physical Well-being Can Change Your Life

Comments from some of the participants indicate that their new-found sense of physical well-being has changed their entire lives. They say their psychological state, their entire outlook, has improved along with their physical condition. There are few scientific data in this subject area to document such a contention, but certainly we are no longer so naive as to believe that mind and body are completely separate entities. Rather, we are coming to realize more and more how intricately interwoven and interdependent a person's mental and physical functions must be. There is no longer much doubt that improved body function also improves the functional state of the mind. Again, consider: "gift of life . . . as long as you are physically and mentally able. . . ."

This brings me to a personal question: What is the state of your health today?

You might answer that you have no problems. Your last medical examination disclosed no disease. So you guess you're in good health. But do you experience a positive sense of physical well-being? Do you have the endurance that makes play enjoyable after a day's work, or are you pooped? Are you able to remain trim, or are you losing the battle of the bulge? Do you sleep well and awaken rested, or do you feel you haven't slept at all? Can you really relax during the day, or is the rat race getting rattier and racier, producing tension? Do you ascend a flight of stairs without undue stress, or do the steps loom like Mount Everest? In short, do you enjoy *positive good health?*

Let's take a moment to clarify our thinking about health. The all-too-prevalent concept defines health simply as the absence of disease. This reasoning says a person who does not have any particular illness is healthy. Not only is this negative in itself; it fails to recognize the *potential* of a person above and beyond the "absence of disease" state. An individual is not usually entirely well, or for that matter, entirely sick. You say you have no illness. But the next question is: How do you feel?

I suggest to you that the scale of health goes not only from disease to "absence of disease," but beyond. It extends onward and upward into the realm of *positive good health,* to the top end of the scale, which would be the vibrant, vigorous good health enjoyed by the well-conditioned athlete. This is what physical fitness is all about.

**Figure 2-1 Positive Health Concept**

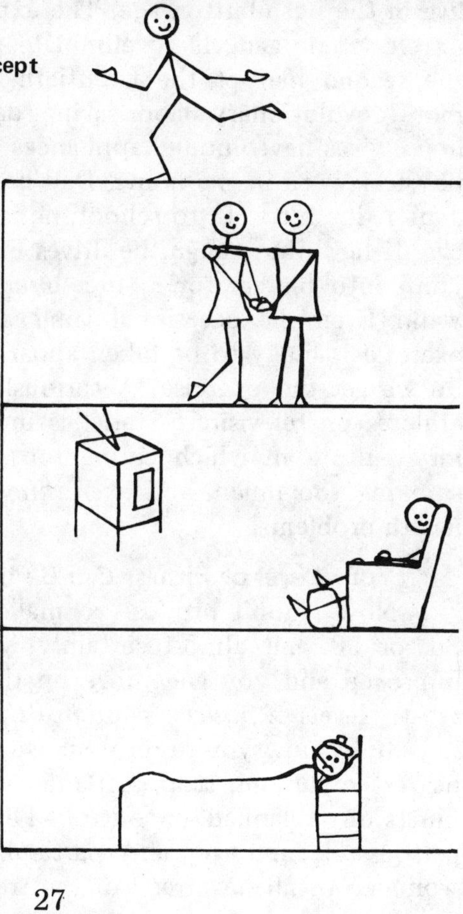

**The well-trained athlete**

**"A" Positive Good Health**

**"B" Absence of Disease**

**"C" Disease**

Figure 2-1 illustrates the positive health concept. The thrust of our research has been to show that controlled, planned exercise can move the normal older person from the B category into the A group of those who enjoy *positive good health:* the physical state in which the individual has the sensation of positive well-being and considerable reserves of energy—in short, vigor!

The unfortunate truth is that most of us have never experienced the sensation of *positive good health*, and, consequently, don't even know it exists. This is because most people today live a less active existence at various phases of life than our forebears. Most of our grandparents regularly performed physical labor of some kind on the farm or in industry. But we live in the push-button age. The explosion of technology, with its electronic gadgets to eliminate physical labor, has molded the second half of the twentieth century and promises even more revolutionary labor-saving devices in the future. Most housewives have enough appliances to reduce or eliminate hard physical work in the home. Dad has a motorized lawn mower. Junior doesn't walk to school; he is driven in the bus or family car. If he's old enough, he drives himself and is more likely to jump into his car for a three-block trip to the store than to walk. Even the occasional jaunt around the golf course for exercise is likely to be taken aboard an electric golf cart. How do we get our exercise? Vicariously, by watching professional athletes on television! Statistics indicate we have a contemporary culture in which eating too much, drinking too much, smoking too much, and *exercising too little* constitute major health problems.

### Your Level of Fitness *Can* Be Improved

Now I don't propose to make athletes of you at age 70, 80, or 90; but almost certainly, your level of fitness can be improved and you can move up the scale toward greater and greater levels of *positive good health.*

If by now you're on your way out the door to climb the nearest mountain, stop. Let me caution you that spontaneous bursts of unplanned, uncontrolled exercise can be hazardous for persons of any age, and particularly for the older man or woman. We all have read of the tragic and unnecessary deaths which occur when persons of middle or advanced age, unaccustomed to vigorous exercise, overstrain themselves. In wintertime, we hear far too often of *John Doe* who for months has done nothing more strenuous than tie his shoelaces, going out to do battle with the snow on his walk. He collapses; perhaps dies. This might have been an unnecessary death, because had he maintained a suitable level of fitness, the snow shoveling might have challenged only a small fraction of his capacity and he would not have overstrained his heart. I should qualify this last statement by adding "in the absence of heart disease."*

Even the conditioning program itself, if unplanned and uncontrolled, can constitute a hazard, especially in the presence of unrecognized heart disease. For these reasons, it appeared to me that we needed a basis for exact prescription of exercise—a book such as the compendium known as the *U.S. Pharmacopoeia,* which the physician has at his disposal for prescribing drugs. What is needed is a book or pharmacopoeia of exercise. In our studies, we took the first few faltering steps in this direction. We asked the questions: (1) How much exercise is enough? (2) How much is too much? and (3) How does one go about putting exercise prescriptions on a sound scientific basis? The results of our work have been published in the medical literature so that your physician will be better able to help you in your conditioning program.[2]

Fortunately, the stress of exercise can be easily measured. In the normal individual, the rise in heart rate during any physical activity is directly proportional to the stress imposed on the heart, lungs, and blood vessels. Using this measure, and correlating such factors as age, physical fitness level, and the type and rate of exercise, we can produce graphs and tables from which an exercise program can be planned. With guesswork eliminated, the program can become an individual plan, designed to produce just enough stress to bring about a beneficial training effect, but not enough to be hazardous in any way. This, in essence, is our "exercise prescription" approach to helping you set up the best possible plan on a "do it yourself" basis.

---

*More on this and the need for a pre-exercise physical in later chapters.

A very important principle that must be used in planning exercise is *progression.* As you condition your body, its capacity for work gradually improves. With time and repeated exercise sessions, the amount of activity which at first was a heavy load becomes too easy. Notice that the word "gradually" is emphasized; it is a key idea. All progress must be gained slowly, at a rate which suits you, personally. Any attempt at too rapid an increase in workload on your system can be hazardous. And purely in practical terms, such an effort is doomed to failure anyway, because the bout then becomes exhausting. It is detrimental instead of providing the stimulus to improvement.

Our work has shown that we need only exercise to between 40 and 60 percent of our capacity to gain the benefits. For unconditioned older people, exercising much harder than that is dangerous and impractical.

Another point that needs emphasis at the outset is that improved physical fitness and consequent vigor are permanent possessions only so long as we continue the "good life" of regular exercise. It takes relatively little exercise to maintain fitness once it is accomplished. But when a person backslides into the completely sedentary life, the previous unfit condition results. When you consider that we have been able to demonstrate such remarkable improvements in the vigor of older persons with an exercise regimen requiring only three hours per week—three out of 112 waking hours of the average person—it appears to be a small investment of time indeed. Many of our enthusiastic subjects say this small investment of time and effort has yielded them a thousandfold profit. *Positive good health*—the joys of being 100 percent alive through improved fitness—has produced the necessary motivation.

### Putting to Rest Some Old Wives' Tales

At this point, let me put to rest some old wives' tales which have been accepted as fact over the years probably because they have been so often repeated. First, there is the old story that exercise causes "athlete's heart." Years ago, before we knew better, the large heart of the athlete was considered to be abnormal because in some types of heart disease the heart becomes greatly enlarged. But now we know that the large heart of the athlete is the result of having developed a stronger, healthier heart muscle. Enlargement of the heart in disease is quite the opposite—it is the result of a weakened, less functional organ, and is part of the ailment itself.

I have heard the saying, "hard work makes you old before your time." That can be true if an individual works to exhaustion day after day throughout his life. But that is quite different from what I'm suggesting to you. Let me quote some of the outstanding scientists in heart disease prevention, Doctors Skinner, Holloszy, and Cureton. They have concluded that a vigorous exercise program "produces changes in functional capacity and body composition that run counter to the trend usually seen with aging."[3]

There are those among us who like exercise best when a machine does all the work. Unfortunately, neither you nor the machine benefits from this sort of activity to any extent. In order to achieve desired conditioning benefits, the exercise must stress your system to a degree. It must make demands on your heart, lungs, and muscles somewhat greater than those to which you have become accustomed in the normal day's living.

Don't misunderstand. I'm *not* saying that if a little exercise is good, a lot must be better. One of our research subjects, 69 years old when he joined our program, was a superbly conditioned man for his age. I realized that we probably could not produce much improvement in him because he was starting at the top, or very near it. At the time he joined our program, he had been bicycling rigorously and playing hard, competitive tennis daily. He continued this regimen even in addition to the exercise prescription we were providing. It was not surprising that at the first re-testing he had not improved. Instead, the double-barreled load had led him to near-exhaustion. Obviously, I advised him against such a heavy exercise schedule. For this man, an exceptional case, any added activity over and above that of his normal lifestyle was undesirable. He already had established exercise patterns which for him were relatively ideal.

### Ours Is a Sensible, Laboratory-tested Program

You will see many advertisements for all sorts of miraculous and magic exercise fads. Science has demonstrated that in health matters, the days of black magic are long gone. There is no magical way to physical fitness. There are only sensible and nonsensical methods. I claim no magic nor even a unique exercise program. What I do have for you is a sensible program which is laboratory-tested and proven to be both safe and effective for older people.* [4]

If you're enthusiastic about the prospects of renewed vigor in your advanced years through exercise, let me caution you again: Don't rush out and run a mile.

To the contrary, the very first "exercise" I prescribe for you at this point is to turn the pages of this book and read all of the following chapters carefully. You will read a nontechnical description of our scientific findings and those of others. There are discussions of the benefits for heart, lungs, and circulation; increases in energy; relaxation from tensions; alleviation of joint stiffness; maintenance of proper body weight; then, the all-important "how to." Included in the latter are the preparations for the program, including the most important safety measure: examination and consultation by your physician.

The fact that you've gotten this far into the book might indicate you're on your way into following in the footsteps of the older persons with whom we've worked.

Like you, perhaps, a few years back they probably never expected that they would be embracing a physically active life for the first time in their mature years. Nor did they expect to gain renewed vigor after retirement age.

They made the wonderful discovery that it was within their power to renew themselves in the basic physical capacities that underlie a full life. So also can you. It is almost a certainty that with this program you can provide yourself a state of *positive good health*—one of the essentials to live, love, laugh, play, work, grow, achieve self-fulfillment, and contribute to the lives of others—as a pioneering citizen of the Nation of the Retired.

---

*Because I do not wish to bore you by belaboring statistics and descriptions of our scientific procedures, I will hold all technical details to a minimum. However, because some of you might wish to read the original data, or have your physician read them, I have included source information for the data in the chapter notes at the end of the book.

# 3

# YOUNG AT HEART . . .

## Cardiovascular-Respiratory Health

Forty million times a year.

That's the number of beats of the average human heart. Each day, with about 100,000 contractions, an average of 2,500 gallons of blood is pumped through this incredible powerhouse. In its operation, the heart services many thousands of miles of blood vessels in the average adult. One researcher has underscored the power of the heart in his calculation that heart muscles work twice as hard as the leg muscles of a person who is running. We can always sit down to rest when our limb and trunk muscles are fatigued but the heart keeps going as long as we live. A phenomenally efficient and durable muscle, the heart gets only a fraction of a second of rest between beats.

It is important to recognize that the heart indeed is a muscle, or more accurately, a group or "package" of muscles, similar in many respects, but not all, to the muscles of our legs and arms. As limb muscles are strengthened and improved by exercise, so also is the heart muscle. Research evidence that exercise enhances heart functioning has been developed over the past several decades.

### A Sampling of Evidence of Enhanced Heart Functioning

- In a widely quoted investigation, Dr. Morris and his colleagues studied bus drivers and conductors of the

London Transit Authority. Among 31,000 drivers and conductors, they found that the drivers suffered significantly more coronary heart disease than the conductors. The drivers might be considered sedentary, while the conductors of the double-decked buses did considerable walking and stair-climbing. It seems reasonable to conclude that the conductors suffered less coronary heart disease precisely because of their greater physical activity.

• In Finland, Dr. Karvonen compared the electrocardiograms of lumberjacks with those of men in less vigorous occupations. He found that abnormalities were only one-fourth as common in the physically active lumberjacks.

• At the University of Minnesota, Dr. Taylor and his colleagues collected data on persons representing nearly 200,000 years (number of subjects times years studied) of heart disease risk. They found more than twice the death rate from heart disease among clerks as compared with more active men.

• The "why and how" for these data are best explained by the classic experiments of Dr. Eckstein, in which he created artificially restricted coronary arteries in dogs by means of surgery. Among these experimental animals, those which were exercised developed significantly better coronary blood flow than ones which were kept sedentary. The exercise seemed to bring about the development of new connections between the impaired vessels and nearly normal blood vessels, so that in the exercised dogs the blood supply was better maintained to all the muscle tissue of the heart.

• Dr. Wilhelm Raab, who was a cardiologist at the Medical College of the University of Vermont, was a leader in the movement to use exercise for the prevention of coronary heart disease. He and his colleagues demonstrated that the combination of coronary blood vessel constriction (plugging with cholesterol) with emotionally excited states brings about electrocardiographic changes typical of coronary heart disease. Responding to our hectic way of life, the endocrine glands and the nervous system pour adrenaline and similar substances into the bloodstream. The presence of these substances in the blood augments the effect of the coronary blood vessel constriction. The effects of exercise, however, are vagotonic. This means that they are opposed to the action of the adrenaline. Consequently, exercise offers some protection against the effects of adrenaline produced by emotions and anxiety.

**Benefits to Those Who Have Had Heart Attacks**

It is interesting to note the impressive benefits which have accrued to the victims of coronary heart disease—those who have had heart attacks—when exercise programs are designed for them. Dr. Gottheiner in Israel, Dr. Hellerstein in Cleveland, and Drs. Kasch and Boyer in San Diego have been leaders in this endeavor. The results have been nothing short of astounding. Men who previously would have been tacitly encouraged to become "cardiac invalids" were in the majority of cases now able to return to pre-heart attack levels of activity. Many of them developed far more vigor than they had before their illness.

In our research, we too have been most concerned with the heart. Our principal focus has been the effects of exercise on heart *function*—how well the heart works. In other words, we asked: Does exercise improve heart function in older people? If so, to what degree? The answers to these questions are important not only for the health of the heart muscle itself, but also because the organ's efficiency is the most important functional element in determining our energy level.

This is so because the heart, as a pump, keeps blood moving throughout the human system. The blood carries life-giving oxygen, which is needed in all active tissues of the body in order to burn foodstuffs to produce energy. In other words, your energy level depends on the availability of oxygen to the active tissues, the muscles. Oxygen supply, then, is the limiting factor which determines the rate at which we can play or work.

Getting oxygen from the air around us to the muscles, which are involved in increased activity, requires the combined and coordinated efforts of several of the body's systems. First, we must move the air from the atmosphere in and out of the lungs to bring it into close contact with the blood, which transports the oxygen to the tissues. And, of course, the rate at which the blood can deliver oxygen to the muscles depends on how well the heart functions as a pump in moving the blood from the lungs to the muscles.

Given then that the heart's functional capacity is the most important element in determining our vigor, we needed a means of measuring heart function to evaluate the effectiveness of our conditioning program. Because of the specifics of our purpose and the advanced age range of our subjects, we were not able to use either of the two best, tried-and-true measurements—those of maximum cardiac output (the heart's capacity to increase blood flow rate) or maximum oxygen consumption. Measurement of maximal cardiac output is a hospital procedure involving the placement of tubes within the heart. Measurement of maximal oxygen consumption is more applicable, in the sense that it is a procedure performed routinely in physiology of exercise laboratories such as ours. The test has the individual either walking on a treadmill or pedaling a stationary bicycle under ever-increasing workloads. But the problem is that this test is useful only on healthy young people, whose muscles are adequate to perform enough work to fully load the heart and circulatory system. In older persons, the procedure would be unnecessarily hazardous. This is because it requires taking the subject to his maximum work level, even slightly beyond, to assure that we have indeed measured his true maximum. Further, our experience in the laboratory has shown that prior to the conditioning program, relatively few older people have enough muscle power to fully load their oxygen transport system.

For these reasons we had to develop laboratory testing techniques better suited to the older individual. That is, we needed a test which could be administered at levels below maximum workload capacity, not only for safety, but also for practicality's sake. Such a test, of course, must provide a reasonably accurate prediction of maximal oxygen consumption. We decided our purpose would be served best by measuring "oxygen-pulse," which is the amount of oxygen consumed per heartbeat. Measured at less strenuous workloads,

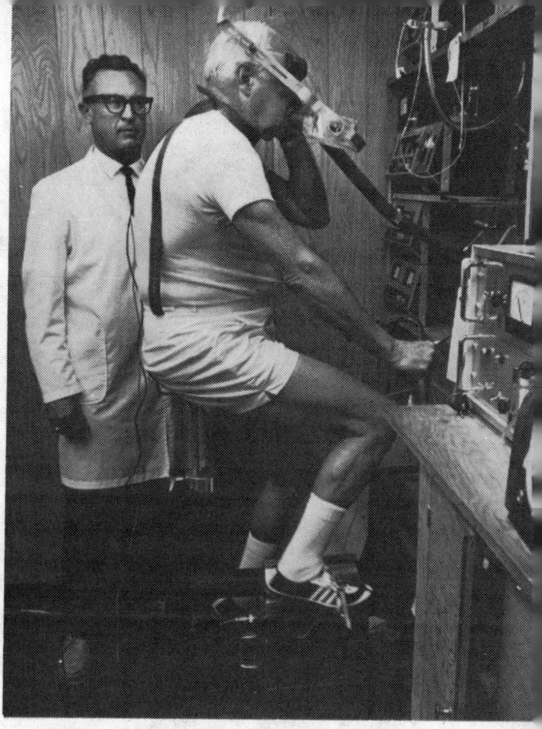

Figure 3-1 Physiological testing is under way as 68-year-old research subject pedals the bicycle ergometer. As subject pedals the apparatus under the watchful eye of Dr. deVries, a whole spectrum of physiological data is being monitored and measured, including electrocardiogram, oxygen consumption, blood pressure, cardiac output and carbon dioxide output. The tension of the pedals can be varied to test physical functions under different levels of stress. (Allan D. Walker)

oxygen-pulse is proportional to maximum oxygen consumption and therefore is a good indicator of it. It is also closely correlated with the stroke volume, that is, the volume of blood pumped by the heart at each contraction (see Figure 3-1).

### A Considerable Renewal in Heart Functioning

The measurement of oxygen-pulse proved to be a successful and efficient method. Importantly, it demonstrated that exercise brought about a considerable renewal in the heart function of our older subjects. That is, despite a chronological age of 60 or 70, many of our subjects' "physiological age" had been reduced. Their hearts were beating and pumping like those of 40- and 50-year-olds. Conservatively speaking, we saw a reduction of 10 to 20 years in their hearts' oxygen transport capacity even if they had been relatively inactive for years. On the average in one study, subjects whom we followed with our testing for 42 weeks improved 29 percent in heart function as measured by oxygen-pulse. Later in the book, we will describe for you an easy home technique to accomplish the same purpose.

In some of our subjects, the improvement was even quite dramatic. R. H., a well-built "young" man of 69, had been in sedentary office work during his career years and had been only moderately active in his leisure time. In the first six weeks of conditioning, his oxygen-pulse improved by 21 percent, and at 42 weeks his improvement had continued to the point that his oxygen-pulse was 42.5 percent better than when he started the exercise program. This probably is not a typical case, however, in that R. H. had been endowed with a rugged constitution, as attested to by his medical history, which showed no significant diseases throughout his life. Now he is an extremely vigorous and healthy looking man in his early seventies.

G. T., age 63, an industrial engineer, had suffered with Hodgkin's disease 11 years earlier and came to our program with a mild reduction in lung capacity, due to radiation treatment. At the start, his oxygen-pulse was one of the lowest we'd seen. By six weeks, he had achieved a level average for his age, and maintained this throughout the 42-week period. His improvement amounted to an impressive 55 percent. We must remember, however, that the lower we start, the greater the potential for improvement.

What do these percentages of improvement mean? When we refer to a 29 percent improvement in oxygen-pulse, we're saying that the heart—with every beat—transports 29 percent more oxygen than it did before. This can be brought home by the often-used example of what happens to the heart rate as the result of an improved oxygen-pulse level. It's a well-known fact that the heart rate—both at rest and during exercise—goes down as the result of physical conditioning. It is typical for the resting heart rate to decrease by at least 10 beats per minute when optimum physical fitness has been attained. Thus, the heart which beats 70 times a minute before training will need to beat 60 or fewer times a minute after several months of conditioning. So instead of 4,200 beats per hour, it's down to 3,600, for a net saving of 14,400 beats in 24 hours. It is precisely because exercise *helps increase the quantity of oxygen* transported by the heart at each beat that the heart needs to beat fewer times a minute to provide oxygen throughout the system. This probably represents a very great reduction of "wear and tear" on your heart.

Under exercise conditions, this saving in heart rate for older people is significant. Take a moderately heavy exercise workload, for example. Let's suppose this given amount of activity will bring the heart rate of a highly conditioned man of 65 up to a comfortable 127 beats per minute. If the same amount of work is attempted by an unconditioned person of the same age, he will probably have to go to his maximum—160 beats per minute or more. In other words, a given amount of work might be a breeze for the older physically fit person, while it would constitute a maximal, "all-out" effort for his poorly conditioned counterpart, with all the accompanying hazards which this implies.

### Improved Breathing

We've discussed the improvements in the heart's ability to move oxygen throughout the system as the result of exercise. Now let's focus for a moment on the most obvious part of oxygen transport, breathing itself. In healthy young people, it is not a lack in breathing capacity that limits physical performance. But what of the older person who for years has been unaccustomed to physical activity? We were struck by the tremendous improvement in breathing capacity in the men who went through our program. On the average, their ability to move large volumes of air in and out of the lungs improved by a surprising 35 percent. The improvements over 42 weeks ranged from a whopping 129 percent in G. T., whose increase in oxygen transport capacity we noted previously, to a mere 15 percent by H. S., who at 52 was the "baby" of the group. H. S.' improvement in breathing capacity, even though the smallest of the group percentagewise, was important. He started the program with a breathing capacity which would be average for a 63-year-old. After 42 weeks, it was average for the 45-year-old range. C. D., 67, started the program with a breathing capacity of a younger man—the 63-year range—yet still improved. At 42 weeks, his capacity was as great as that of a person of 50. H. C., age 69, started at the level of a 75-year-old and improved to the mean for age 62. Again, in terms of breathing, the men had lopped years off their "physiological age." They were breathing much younger.

In breathing capacity, however, there is a marked difference between the sexes. Considering that the men we studied showed such marked improvement, it was surprising to us that women we studied in another experiment showed little or no change in their breathing capacity. In most respects, our female program participants showed training improvements very similar to those of the men. The women's average improvement in oxygen-pulse was 19 percent, not so large as that of the men, who improved 29 percent, but significant nonetheless.

The most likely explanation of this difference between men and women lies in the gradual stiffening of the chest wall due to aging. Research indicates that in men the chest wall tends to lose its elasticity with advancing years. But in women there may be little or no change. As the chest wall stiffens gradually, it creates its own resistance against vigorous breathing. There is reason to believe that agewise loss of elasticity of connective tissues is much greater in the male than in the female. In a recent study using newly developed electronic techniques to measure finger joint stiffness, no real change was found in women between the ages of 50 and 70, compared to women in their twenties. In men, however, the same comparison showed significant decrease of elasticity with increasing age.[1] This suggests that the improvements in breathing capacity registered by our male participants resulted from improving the elasticity of the chest wall, thereby enabling them to breathe more deeply. It is borne out by the fact that the men improved their vital capacity (the greatest volume of air an individual can expel in one breath) while the women did not.

By now, having discussed some of the exercise-induced improvements in the cardiovascular system of older people, hopefully you can see why this chapter is titled "Young at Heart." We've seen how physical conditioning can improve breathing, the first step in the process of supplying oxygen to the tissues of the body. We've also reported our findings of increased efficiency in the second step—the heart's function as a pump in transporting the oxygen throughout the system. Now let's look at the other half of step two—the blood which carries the oxygen. Specifically, let's discuss blood *pressure.*

### The Importance of Blood Pressure

In this health-conscious era, most people are very well aware of the importance of blood pressure to their health.

Blood pressure has aptly been called the "barometer" of health. It can help forecast a person's health much like actual barometers aid in forecasting the weather. The national statistics show clear-cut relationships between high blood pressure, more accurately called hypertension, and disease. Statistical data also demonstrate a definite trend toward high blood pressure with increasing age—at least in our culture, which is undergoing great changes that produce psychological-social stress.[2] It seems unfortunate, indeed, that blood pressure should be the highest at the point in life when our blood vessels are probably least able to withstand the increase.

Have you ever asked yourself why your doctor is so concerned about your blood pressure? You probably have contented yourself with the answer that, just as with an automobile tire, if the pressure is too high, the danger of a "blowout" is greater. The human "blowout" is a stroke or aneurysm. Reason enough, but there are other equally important high blood pressure effects that are not so well known to laymen.

Remember that the heart functions as a pump. As with any pump, energy demands can be increased in two ways: (1) by requiring it to provide a greater flow rate; and (2) by increasing the pressure in the pipes through which the flow circulates. Consider, for example, a pump which is moving water through a closed circuit of pipes, all of which lie at the same level as the pump. If we require the liquid to flow *faster*, we have increased the work the pump must do. Now, let's keep the *flow rate constant*, and increase the work on the pump in a different way: We insert into the circuit of pipes a valve which restricts the flow, thus causing *greater pressure* for the pump to work against. Thus, we have put a greater workload on the pump, while the *flow rate* is unchanged. This sort of experiment has been performed using the heart as the pump. The results showed very clearly that while the heart is not strained at all by requiring of it faster and faster flow rates, the strain does increase very rapidly when the blood pressure is increased. Therefore, high blood pressure is damaging because it puts additional strain on the heart. Complicating this strain is the fact that it is not merely a "sometimes" thing. If blood pressure is chronically too high, the added strain on the heart is constant, 24 hours a day.

Increased blood pressure also can create problems by damaging the interior blood vessel walls, making them more likely to become clogged up. Clogging causes a "coronary" if it occurs in a blood vessel which supplies the heart with blood. If it happens in the brain, the result is a stroke.

Restriction of flow in the blood vessels in hypertension can occur in several ways, such as "plugging up" with fatty deposits, which is called atherosclerosis; by increased activity of the sympathetic nervous sytem, the "fight or flight" system which is activated whenever we are angry, fearful, or anxious; or by abnormal secretions of hormones.

### Significant Improvement in Blood Pressure

Happily, one of the most important changes we saw in our older subjects when we improved their physical fitness level was a significant drop in blood pressure, especially if it had been above normal at the start. As we noted previously, our research subjects were chosen for their basically good health, so most of them had blood pressure readings normal for their ages. The fact that even relatively normal blood pressure can be reduced is significant. On the group average, we saw a 2.4 percent reduction in the systolic (contraction phase of the heartbeat) blood pressure. This was accompanied by a 4.5 percent drop in diastolic (resting phase of the heartbeat) blood pressure. These are not large decreases; but we did not expect huge percentage changes. Drs. Boyer and Kasch showed even greater improvements when subjects started with high blood pressure.[3]

Let's take another brief look, in summary, at what the scientific evidence indicates about the benefits of exercise for the cardiovascular and respiratory systems.

In experiments with animals, it has been shown that when the coronary arteries have been surgically narrowed to simulate the effects of atherosclerosis (deposits of fatty materials which plug up the arteries)[4] and the animals were then given an exercise regimen, better coronary blood flow to the heart muscle resulted. If such results can be said to be applicable to humans, then we might assume the same results: that appropriate exercise regimens can improve blood flow to the heart's muscle tissue, thus resulting in both a smaller likelihood of a heart attack and less severe consequences if a coronary should occur. However, because such experiments are extremely difficult to conduct on humans, direct evidence still is inconclusive. Medical scientists who take a more conservative approach are not yet willing to make such statements with respect to the human. The case for exercise probably is best stated by Dr. Sam Fox, chief of the Heart Disease and Stroke Control Program of the U.S. Public Health Service: ". . . I believe we can consider it highly prudent to include programs of increased habitual activity in our multi-factorial approach to the prevention of coronary heart disease."[5]

### Five Ways the Program Improves Health

I believe it is fair to say that physical conditioning through a careful, well-planned exercise program can be expected to improve the health of the cardiovascular system through several routes. Most importantly, it improves the heart muscle itself. Secondly, it reduces the blood pressure load against which the heart must work 24 hours a day. Third, as we shall see in a later chapter, appropriate exercises in moderation can reduce the tension level in nervous persons.[6] This in turn, helps to normalize blood pressure. Fourth, vigorous exercise helps decrease the percentage of body fat, which reduces the statistical probability of heart attack as well as other diseases. Last, but definitely not least important, an exercise program seems to improve greatly the ability to breathe deeply and efficiently, at least in the older male.

It should be added that physical exercise is a *natural* way of enhancing the health. Uncomplicated by adverse side effects, it improves the body's own regulatory functions. It can help you to become and to remain "Young at Heart."

# 4
# PEP UP!
## Conquering Fatigue

"Doctor, I tire so easily. . . ." "Doctor, I'm always dragging. . . ." "Doctor, I just don't seem to have any energy anymore. . . ."

My physician friends tell me these are the sorts of complaints they hear frequently from their older patients. More often than not, regardless of the primary reason they visit the doctor, the older persons complain of persistent fatigue.

For a contrast, listen to some of our program participants: "I could tell a real difference. . . ." "I can do things now that were a real struggle before. . . ." "I have more get-up-and-go. . . ." "I have more energy. . . ." "I feel more alive. . . ."

### More Energy—Less Fatigue

When we ask our exercisers what they feel the most important results of the conditioning program are for them, the most commonly heard answer is "more energy—less fatigue." J. M. H., age 74, says he no longer tires so easily. R. H., 70, who admits he could not have run at all without difficulty prior to the exercise project, now not only runs, but runs freely and easily, tiring far less quickly than before. Dr. C. H. J., a 71-year-old retired dentist, found that he fatigues less easily than before the conditioning program. These are not isolated cases. Others talk enthusiastically of more energy not only for carrying on normal daily activities but also for pursuit of new and different interests.

How do we account for this relief from fatigue and tiredness brought about by a better level of physical fitness? There are several factors to explain the energy renewal. We discussed the first in the previous chapter. It's that life-giving element, oxygen.

We explained the process by which oxygen is transported from the environment throughout the human system: It is breathed into the lungs, where it links up with the blood, which is pumped by the heart throughout the body. We showed that improved fitness through exercise makes this complex process easier and more efficient. Greater quantities of oxygen are thus available just where the vital substance is needed—at each muscle of the body. We pointed out that a person's energy level depends on this very factor—the availability of oxygen to the active tissues.

Why is this so? Because vigorous physical activity can be sustained only a minute or two without oxygen. Oxygen is a necessary factor for the burning of foodstuffs stored in the muscles, which must occur if vigorous activity lasts more than a couple of minutes. Any prolonged action of any muscle of the body depends on this process of oxidation to generate any unit of energy. Any move you make—whether it is wiggling the index finger, using the large leg muscles in running, or the long arm muscles in playing tennis—depends on the availability of oxygen at the point where the power to move is being generated—in the muscles themselves. You must burn foodstuffs stored in the muscles or supplied by the blood to produce energy. And you must have oxygen "on the spot" to burn the foodstuffs.

The process of burning foodstuffs in the body can be compared to that of burning logs in a fireplace. You cannot start a fire in a vacuum. Even if you were to stack the finest logs in the most expert way and add ample kindling, you would not be able to get a fire going if there were not sufficient oxygen present. On the other hand, if there is plenty of oxygen circulating it is easy to kindle a lively blaze. The more oxygen present at the point of burning, the brighter and hotter the fire will be. It is much the same circumstance in the burning of fuel stored in the muscles to produce energy. Oxygen must get to the point where it is needed and it must be available for the burning of the stored fuel. Generally speaking, as more energy is needed, more foodstuff must be consumed to produce it, and more oxygen is needed to burn this fuel. Thus, the importance of oxygen for increasing a person's energy level.

But that is only half the story. What about the fuel, the stored foodstuff, itself?

We all know that the food we eat becomes fuel. We also are aware that a balanced diet includes different types of foods from three major groupings—proteins, fats, and carbohydrates—as well as "auxiliary foodstuffs,," vitamins, and minerals. Proteins and fats are derived principally from the meat and dairy products categories. Carbohydrates come from bread, grains, and other starchy and sugar foods. We know that each of these foods has specific nourishment roles to play in maintaining our existence. It requires a surprising degree of energy production and dynamic activity in the cells of the body for a person simply to survive.

But what primarily concerns us here is the energy necessary for activities above and beyond mere survival—activities ranging from standing still, through walking, to more strenuous pursuits such as bicycling. Which foods, which fuels are necessary for energy when we bring our muscles into play?

Of the three principal foodstuffs, it has long been known that protein is not normally used as a supply of energy. Fat, broken down to free fatty acids, can be used as an energy source, but it is not the primary fuel for muscle work.

The foodstuff which makes heavier activities possible is a substance called glycogen. This is a complex carbohydrate derived from certain foods we eat, processed by the body and stored in the liver and muscle tissues. Glycogen is the fuel which is "kept on hand" by the muscle to be used when the muscle is called on to produce energy. The supply of glycogen determines and limits the amount of our vigorous activity.

Now, what happens when we exercise vigorously? The activity depletes the glycogen, as this fuel is burned to produce the required energy. But the key point here is this: The exercise causes the level of glycogen *to be replenished in greater quantities* than before. It has been found that when muscle glycogen is depleted by vigorous exercise, the level stored *increases to approximately double* its previous quantity within about three days on a high carbohydrate diet. In contrast, studies have shown that unused muscles do not change their level of glycogen content.[1] Here is one of the more interesting double-pronged effects of a training program: (1) The fuel stored in the muscles is increased. This level of fuel determines the *endurance* of muscle tissue. (2) The oxygen supply is increased and more readily available to the active muscles. This availability of oxygen determines the upper limits of *intensity* of exercise we can sustain.

In other words, exercise not only helps provide more fuel for our physical activities. It simultaneously allows us to burn this fuel at a higher rate, thus allowing more intense activity.

Another factor involved in improving resistance to fatigue (and probably also related to glycogen storage) involves the *amount of muscle tissue* required to work over long periods of time. Through daily experience, everyone knows that sustained vigorous activity produces fatigue. What is not so well known, however, is that the fatigue process results in each muscle fiber producing less force. Hence, more units of muscle must be called into play to get the job done. In our laboratory, using electromyography, a technique requiring complex electronic instrumentation, we have been able to study this process. We found that the better conditioned the muscle is, the slower the rate of recruitment of additional muscle fibers to sustain physical activity.[2] Here's the point: Exercise produces better conditioned muscles; better conditioned muscles require less of themselves to perform work.

A person who is not engaged in much hard physical activity during the course of the day might question how this point can be part of the anwer to his or her fatigue problems. Let me point out to you that unless you're flat on your back, your muscles are working all day long. They might even be working to some degree when you are lying down if you're a tense person. For example, we have examined the nature of fatigue that occurs in the muscles of the lower back when a person is doing nothing more strenuous than simply standing still in the most relaxed fashion possible.[3] We have seen clear evidence of this fatigue process in some of our subjects. Just the energy requirements of standing still taxed some of their lower back muscle fibers to the point that more units of muscle had to be brought into play. Interestingly, only the individuals who developed low back pain from prolonged standing (22 minutes) showed evidence of fatigue. What I am saying to you in essence, then, is that no heroic efforts are required in producing muscle fatigue if the muscles are in poor condition to begin with. Seemingly simple and easy muscle activity such as standing, walking, or even sitting can bring about fatigue if the muscles are sufficiently debilitated.

The happy aspect of all this is that muscle function can be improved by appropriate exercise at any age. In the absence of disease, the improvement is greatest in persons with poorer strength levels at the start.

Here's another way of looking at this problem of fatigue. Let's use a concrete example: You and your neighbor are going to take a bicycle ride at 10 miles per hour. Let's say that 10 mph is as fast as you can go, but your neighbor is capable of 20 mph. In this situation, you will be able to continue only half as long as your neighbor. Looking at it another way, if you stop at some point well within your capacity, your neighbor will be only half so fatigued as you. Thus, the better your physical working capacity, other things being equal, the slower your rate of fatigue (see Figure 4-1).

**Figure 4-1 Are you peppy . . . or do you just drag along?**

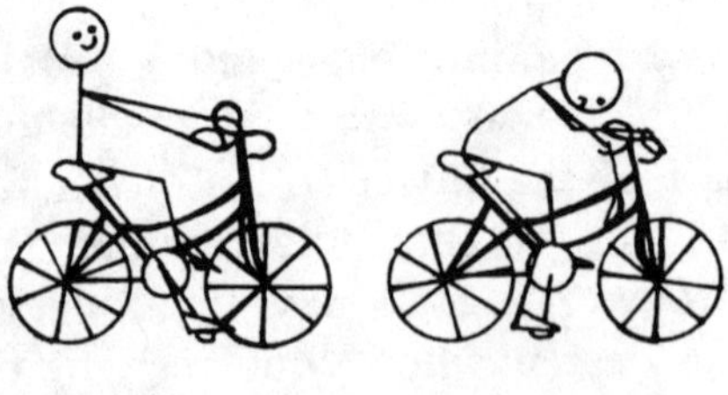

In our laboratory, we measure physical working capacity in many ways. One that is easily understood by our participants is to put them on our stationary bicycle and raise the workload every two minutes until we get to approximately 85 percent of their maximal heart rate. The total work accomplished up to this point is an excellent criterion of how rapidly they fatigue.

Our retired dentist, Dr. C. H. J., was able to produce 513 watt minutes of work at a heart rate of 145 when he started our conditioning program. After 42 weeks of training, he had increased his capacity so that when his heart rate hit 145, he had completed 760 watt minutes of work. This represents a net gain of 48 percent in his physical work capacity. Small wonder that he, like many others, is delighted with his new-found pep!

# 5

# RE-L-A-X-X-X

# Eliminating Nervous Tension

Uptight.

We have the younger generation to thank for coining this interesting expression. My friends who are knowledgeable about slang tell me the word can have a variety of shadings and connotations, but one of its main uses is as a crisp, crackling, slap-in-the-ear description of a person who is nervous and tense. "Uptight" conjures up all sorts of images, such as an over-stressed guitar string or an over-wound watch—both nearing the breaking point. Importantly for our purposes here, the word graphically conveys the concept of nervous tension. It is apparent that nervous tension is one of the major problems of our society today. Far too many Americans are uptight.

Americans spend vast amounts of money each year for drugs to relieve tension, ranging from over-the-counter sleeping pills to prescribed tranquilizers. The importance of nervous tension as a health problem is beyond dispute.

## The Effect of Nervous Tension on Our Health

The role of nervous tension in various diseases has been investigated by Dr. Edmund Jacobson, who also pioneered in the scientific measurement of tension. As early as the 1920s and the 1930s, Jacobson already had suggested some of the relationships between nervous tension and disease.[1] He gained vast experience in applying his relaxation methods to various ailments for which his patients consulted him. This provided considerable evidence that many health problems could be lessened—if not completely cured—if the patient could be taught to relax away his nervous tension.

Jacobson's reports to many medical journals and the case histories contained in his early books showed the beneficial effects of relaxation in such ills as asthma, insomnia, high blood pressure, neuroses, neurasthenia, and some disorders of the stomach and colon. In case after case, he was able to show the damaging effects of unnecessary nervous tension. Importantly, he was able to bring about relief through teaching his patients to relax. The effects of their new-found relaxation were parlayed through the various systems of the body.

Other scientific investigators have followed Jacobson's lead. Over the years, a considerable body of scientific knowledge has been developed substantiating the undesirable effects of unnecessary nervous tension on human health. This is particularly true in the areas of psychiatry and psychosomatic medicine.[2]

The effect of nervous tension on our health is a rather insidious one, because until the problem is quite severe, we are unlikely to recognize the symptoms. The early symptoms, such as "jitteriness," insomnia, irritability, easy fatigue, and headaches, are apt to come on slowly and progressively. They are not recognized to be real threats to health until they are well established.

What exactly is this disturber and complicator of life and health called "nervous tension"? In general, it's the result of our increasingly strident combat with our environment. It is abundantly obvious that our cultural transformation just in the last century in this country has complicated our lives as sensing, thinking beings. The conversion from a relatively peaceful agricultural-frontier mode of living to the highly complex, fast-paced, crowded, and intense existence most of us lead in the space-age megalopolis has been accompanied by a rapidly increasing overload on our nervous systems.

The human nervous system is a wonderful complex network which underlies the vast number of functions—such as sensing, moving, thinking, reacting—that we tend to take for granted in the course of our daily lives. This marvelously integrated and normally efficient system is responsible in many ways for our survival.

Interestingly, a certain amount of what we call tension is necessary in the proper operation of the human system. When we pick up a book for example, the action is the result of a series of lightning-fast functions. The brain signals the arm, wrist, and hand muscles to contract in certain ways to pick up the book. In the contraction of the muscles, a certain amount of tension has been generated. So a certain amount of tension is necessary for us to function as humans. But too much nervous tension is destructive to us. The same principle of enough versus excess can be seen operating in other systems and organs of the body. Take the hydrochloric acid of the stomach, for example. A normal level of this chemical is essential for digestion, as we all know. But excess amounts of it can cause ulcers. Like the stomach, the nervous system operates on a delicate balance. Enough tension is good and necessary. Too much can be disastrous. When the latter occurs, you have the destructive state of what we call nervous tension, or what the younger generation aptly describes as being "uptight."

How does a person become nervous and tense? Nervous tension can arise at any point in the complex nervous system. It comes about in different ways in different individuals, and victims of nervous tension vary greatly in their responses and symptoms. For the sake of discussion, let's consider excess nervous tension in terms of external causes and internal causes. Both can contribute to nervous tension singly or simultaneously. Nervous tension can be the result of overstimulation of the senses by the environment, and it can arise internally from mental stress.

You have only to look around to see immediately how our senses can become overtaxed and battered by our space-age surroundings. City noise—from traffic, aircraft, blaring radio and television sets, you name it—pummels our ears. Smog assaults our eyes and noses. Urban overcrowding tends to concentrate, accentuate, and augment this multifaceted harangue of our senses.

In addition to the sensory overkill we're subjected to, our pace of life all too easily can produce mental stress, worry, and anxiety, which lead to nervous tension. We are pressured in our jobs by competition, or by the need to perform at a certain level, sometimes with the additional aggravation of a time deadline. Everything has to be done now, today. Mañana is not soon enough for us. Changes in society are coming faster now, perhaps, than at any time in history. We are pressured to adapt. We are pressured to be or not to be; to buy or not to buy; to do or not to do; to conform or not to conform.

Overstimulation of the senses and mental stress frequently combine to cause nervous tension, and there's probably no more common way of experiencing this than driving on today's frantic freeways and expressways. All the operations of driving at high speeds require constant sensory observations, rapid-fire decisions and some guesswork about what the other drivers are going to do. Did you ever stop to consider the extent to which the senses are constantly involved in this nerve-wrenching operation? Add to this the anxiety that can result from the need to be constantly alert, and you can understand why you might arrive at your destination still tense, or physically and mentally "wrung out" from being tense during the drive.

In order to understand how the mental and physical barrage on our nervous system affects us, let's consider a simple reflex, the "startle reflex." If someone shoots off a firecracker in a crowd, the responses of the individuals will vary from mild annoyance to near hysteria. Further, the effect in any one individual will vary from day to day. On the day when a person has worked under relatively serene conditions, he might react to the firecracker with equanimity. However, if the person has been working under the additional strain of jackhammer noise all day, the same firecracker explosion might cause a wild jump, or even tears.

These differences are due to a phenomenon of nerve physiology called the "all or none" law. That is, every nerve cell, or neuron, either responds to its maximum capability, or not at all. It could be compared to a firearm. The nerve cell, like the rifle, either fires, or it doesn't fire. But here's the rub: Nerve cells can be stimulated by sensory information or by mental stress to change from a quiet state to a potentially active one. This is similar to the situation that exists when the safety switch on a rifle is turned off. If the weapon is dropped or jarred, it may fire. When many of the nerve cells throughout our body have been overstimulated all day, either "internally" from mental stress or "externally" from sensory overkill, the cells are near the point of "firing" too. That is, they are on the threshold of firing off impulses to the brain. If even a slight further stimulus occurs, it may set off many of the nerve cells at once, literally bombarding the central nervous system. Such a condition can be compared to the massive snarl which might result in a telephone system if everyone decided to place a long-distance call through the operator at the same time.

And this tension "snarl" of the nervous system is even worse than it appears, because it brings about a vicious cycle. The more active the central nervous system is, the likelier it is to become even more active. This is so because of a "feedback" mechanism of what we call "sensory receptors" in the muscles. These receptors feed back to the central nervous system information on what the muscles are doing. This information is necessary; without it, no coordinated movement would be possible. But the system is so set up that the more active the central nervous system is because of the bombardment we described, the more sensitive and active these sensory receptors in the muscles become. Therefore, with more activity from the receptors, all the more sensory information comes into the central nervous sytem. This is why muscle receptor involvement in nervous tension is so often perceived as muscle tension, and why stiff, uncoordinated movement often results when a person is "tense." However, this same phenomenon results in our ability to measure"nervousness," and also to bring about some degree of control over it, as we shall see.

Because of nervous tension's threat to health, science needed sensitive and objective means of measurement to study causal relationships between tension and disease and to evaluate therapeutic effects of relaxation training. Jacobson recognized this, and with the help of Bell Telephone Laboratories engineers, he developed electronic instruments for measurement and recording of the electrical changes in muscle when it is activated. These minute electrical changes are an indicator of the tension level. They accompany any activity of muscle, even when the activity cannot be discerned by the observer, and what is more important, even when the individual himself is completely unaware there is nervous activation of his muscles. In fact, these electrical changes occur at any time the nervous system sends impulses to the muscles, even when the muscles are totally incapable of response, as in complete fatigue. Consequently, the measurement of the electrical changes in muscles furnishes an opportunity to evaluate the activity of the nervous system when the individual is supposedly at rest.

### Improvement in Participants' Ability to Relax

Putting these electronic methods to work in our laboratory, we performed routine tests of nervous tension in the subjects participating in our study of exercise sponsored by the Administration on Aging. It was intriguing to us that despite the fact that our subjects had been chosen for their good health, we nevertheless saw improvements in their ability to relax as they improved their physical condition.

For some, improved ability to relax was one of the most important effects of our exercise program. Such was the case for C.D., 68, who had spent his professional life as a manufacturing jeweler. The tension-creating tasks of operating his business in the face of stiff competition, coupled with virtually complete physical inactivity during most of his life, were taking their toll as he reached retirement age. For years, he had suffered from very severe tension headaches on the average of three and four times a week. He admits he "ate aspirin like peanuts" for relief. As a magazine writer who later interviewed him described it, C.D. "felt as tense inside as a tightly-wound watch."

When he started the exercise program, our tests disclosed that the electrical activity in his muscles was higher than average, indicating that he was tense and unable to relax as well as he might. After five months of physical conditioning, his muscular electrical activity was down to 37 percent of what it had been, and he no longer had migraine headaches. Interestingly, he went on a motoring vacation at this point, and after ten days of traveling without exercising, his headaches returned with their previous severity. For the remainder of his vacation, he exercised as best he could, and again gained virtually complete relief from his headaches. As a scientist, I cannot claim that we have a cure for all headaches. But I can say that this is what happened for one man (it has since happened for others), and it suggests that for some people, at least, physical conditioning might provide relief from tension-induced headaches.

On the average, our experimental exercising subjects reduced their resting muscle activity by about 10 percent, in spite of its having been relatively low at the start. When these data were compared with data from a previous experiment with university faculty, it was interesting to note that our older exercise subjects started the program with tension-level scores that were less than half the average for the younger university group. Whether this lower tension level represents an effect of aging in itself, or reflects the differences between active professional life and retirement, we cannot say at this point.

In any event, I was struck by the potential value of exercise as a tranquilizer for the older age group. It has long been known that as people grow older, their reaction times are not so fast and their movements are slower. This slowness renders older people particularly vulnerable as drivers, pilots, and even as pedestrians. If we add to the natural slowing effect of aging the additional slowing effect of any of the tranquilizer drugs, we have set up a potentially lethal situation. For this reason, we thought it worthwhile to conduct an additional study of relaxation in older people. We solicited the participation of highly nervous patients from the Laguna Hills Leisure World Medical Center and others from the community. Each subject acted as his own control in that he was exposed to five different experimental treatments: (1) control, (2) tranquilizer drug, (3) placebo, (4) 15 minutes' exercise at a heart rate of 100, (5) 15 minutes' exercise at a heart rate of 120. We found that neither single doses of tranquilizer nor placebo had any significant effect on the ability to relax. But the average effect of the exercise dose was a highly significant reduction of electrical muscle activity ranging from 20 to 25 percent for at least an hour and a half after the exercise.[3] The exercise we administered was the laboratory equivalent of a brisk, 15-minute walk. In other words, even a brisk walk, a relatively mild form of exercise, is significantly effective in relaxing a person, while a single tranquilizer pill is not. This is not to say that tranquilizer drugs are not effective in larger doses and when taken over a period of time. They are effective, of course. But it is precisely under such conditions that the slowing of reactions would be most severe in older people, and cause the most serious potential hazard.

Those of you with a more scientific bent might ask: How, exactly, is this tranquilizer effect brought about by exercise? We are not yet certain. But we do know that in experiments with cats, raising the temperature of either the muscle receptors or the part of the brain called the hypothalamus reduces the activity of the muscle receptors and thereby brings about relaxation to the point of drowsiness. Vigorous exercise is accompanied by such a rise in temperature. Investigators in this scientific area also have suggested that moving the muscles, as is done in exercise, is necessary to keep the muscle receptors' transmissions at a normal level. In contrast, more-or-less constant tightening up of the muscles such as occurs in nervous tension brings about a chronic overactivity in the arousal of the brain. This in turn generates apprehension, fear, and other "tense" emotions.[4]

### The Case for Developing the Ability to Relax

To summarize, here's the case for developing the ability to relax: While all the evidence is not in, the available knowledge indicates that the well-relaxed individual: (1) works more efficiently, (2) thinks more clearly, (3) finds less need for tranquilizers and stimulants, and (4), in general, has fewer health problems related to tension, such as headaches and high blood pressure. In the last ten years, we have conducted five different studies on young, middle-aged, and older men and women in which appropriate exercise has been shown to improve the ability to relax both immediately and over a sustained period. This is another indication to us of the desirability of controlled exercise—all its "side effects" are beneficial.

The moral of this story, then, is: Exercise and RE—L——A———X————X—————X.

# 6

# WHAT'S A JOINT LIKE THAT DOING IN A NICE PERSON LIKE YOU?

## Alleviating Joint Stiffness

You're walking down the street at twilight. At about 200 feet distant, you perceive the figure of a man. The light is poor, providing little more than a silhouette of the figure ahead of you. Nevertheless, you're able to tell he's an older man. How did you know that? You weren't close enough to see familiar indications of aging, such as skin changes or gray hair. In all likelihood, you observed a stooped posture or a slow, shortened stride. These were the signs which told you he was an older man.

I am happy to report, however, that these all-too-common changes in posture and gait do not necessarily have to accompany the aging process, provided the person does not suffer from a significant disease of the joints. I can show you many men in their eighties, who by virtue of the vigorous life and its resultant physical fitness, still stand and walk erect and have a youthful spring in their stride. Indeed, I can point with pride to 80-plus-year-olds who not only walk well, but run and swim in youthful form.

Many limitations of posture and movement caused by joint stiffness are akin to the proverbial gate that is difficult to open and close because of a rusty hinge. Through disuse, the hinge has become balky and stiff. As with most physiological functions, use begets improvement, whereas disuse results in dysfunction. If we don't move our joints throughout all possible ranges of motion, we will lose some of their potential for movement. As a result we are faced with another one of those vicious cycles: Lack of movement over prolonged periods, as we've said, causes the joint to lose its range of motion. This loss causes pain when an attempt is made to move the joint. And pain is a great discourager of further efforts to move.

We can see this cycle occurring to some extent when persons of any age suffer a broken leg which requires the application of a cast and consequent immobilization. When the cast comes off, the patient has a very stiff knee joint. Bad enough that he has temporarily lost so much of his joint motion range; but to complicate the predicament, the much-needed therapy of movement is inhibited by the pain, causing the person to minimize his use of the knee. This avoidance of moving the joint only tends to further restrict movement.

It is an established fact that when a muscle is not at least occasionally worked through its normal range of movement that muscle becomes shortened, often producing spasms and cramps which can be simply irritating or severely painful.

But hold on here, you say. This discussion was to be about joints, not muscles. So it was and so it is: Only recently, a series of experiments at Johns Hopkins Medical School was reported[1] in which it was shown that *joint stiffness probably resides primarily in the muscles and connective tissues that serve to move the joints, rather than in the joint structure itself.*

At Johns Hopkins, Drs. Johns and Wright conducted a study of wrist flexing and extending in the cat, very similar functionally to that in man. Their findings apply directly only to the wrist joint, but undoubtedly their data go far in explaining the problem in other joints as well.

Briefly, they found that the most important factors limiting the range of joint motion are the muscles (including their "sheaths" called fascia), the joint capsule, and the tendons. They further discovered that frictional resistance generated by the two rubbing surfaces of bones in the joint is negligible. This appears to be true even for joints that have been damaged by arthritis.

Let's take a moment to look at the anatomy and physiology involved so that you will better understand the "stiffening up" process that most of us accept as we grow older.

**The Quality of Flexibility**

The range of joint motion from full movement in one direction to full movement in the other is often referred to as the quality of flexibility. The greater the range of motion, the more flexible the individual is in that particular joint. Equally important as the measurable angular range of joint motion are the dynamic qualities of movement. They have to do with the force and energy required to move the joint. In other words, it is one thing to be able to achieve a full bend forward at the hips in order to touch your toes with your fingertips. This is a measure of range of motion. But it is an entirely different matter to be able to make such movements with a minimum of force and expenditure of energy—to move easily and loosely, as it were.

Now, what sets the limits of flexibility in terms of range of motion? For some joints, the bony structure sets a definite limit. For example, extension of the elbow joint and the knee joint are regulated in this fashion. Also, in a very heavily muscled person, it is likely that flexing of his elbow and knee joints would be limited by the bulk of the intervening muscle. These are mechanical factors that cannot be greatly modified, and therefore are only of general interest to us.

In such joints as the ankle or hip or back, however, the limitation of motion range is imposed by the soft tissues, the muscles and connective tissues, as we've seen. This then is where our concern lies, because these factors are modifiable by physical methods, and are important in the prevention of aches and pains.

Let's look further at the role of the soft tissues in determining flexibility. Connective tissue, as the name implies, is the tissue that "holds us all together." It binds muscles to bones by *tendons;* binds bone to bone by *ligaments;* and covers and unites muscles with *fascia.* In general, connective tissue forms a framework for all the organs and for the body as a whole. It is these tendons, ligaments, and fascia which grow less extensible with age and thus convey the impression of stiffness.

There has been some very interesting research into the aging of connective tissues. For example, in animal experiments it has been shown that biochemical changes in the tissues which typically accompany aging also can be brought about by *immobilization.* These findings point to the importance of physical activity in the maintenance of normally functioning connective tissues.[2]

To further emphasize the importance of the connective tissues, it has been pointed out that all the cells of the body (except those floating free in the blood) are ultimately dependent upon the integrity of the connective tissues in order that their energy-producing processes may continue uninterrupted. This is because oxygen and nutrients must reach the cells by way of the connective tissues. Accordingly, it is hypothesized that these tissues may play a key role in aging by their influence on the transport of nutrients and the products of metabolism into and out of the cells.[3]

But more to our point here: Of the three important types of connective tissues, the tendons probably are the most difficult to stretch because their fibers are so densely packed. Ligaments are less difficult to stretch. The muscle fascia, or "sheaths," probably give us the best opportunity to stretch to improve joint mobility.

It is widely believed also that muscle fascia becomes increasingly susceptible to shortening as a function of aging and/or lack or exercise.[4] This shortening places undue pressure on nerve pathways located in the fascia. The result is that many aches and pains are the result of nerve impulses traveling along the already pressured pathways.

This is even worse than it sounds because when muscle pain occurs, it brings about a "splinting reflex" which is designed to immobilize the muscle by making it contract. But the further contraction only serves to shorten the connective tissues again. This brings about a vicious cycle which results in tying up the whole area involved in the muscle spasm. The typical low-back pain syndrome is one of the most common results of this kind of cycle.

We have conducted a series of studies in my laboratory directed to this problem. We used highly sensitive electromyography instrumentation which was designed and built for us for this specific purpose. The experiments were carried on over a five-year period and results have been published in scientific journals. A summary for the scientifically oriented reader is available in the *American Journal of Physical Medicine.*[5]

For our study of how muscle pain comes about, we had special research subjects referred to our laboratory. These were persons who were suffering muscle pain brought about by athletic injuries. We made measurements to determine the amount of electrical activity present in the muscle. This is important because the normal, well-relaxed muscle produces no electrical activity. But a muscle in spasm or one that is incompletely relaxed because of pain shows considerable electrical activity due to irritation.

Then, we applied static stretching procedures which long have been known to be effective in relieving cramps. (These are basically the same static stretching exercises you will be provided with in Chapter 9.)

### Stretching Actually Relieves Pain

After the stretching, we remeasured the electrical activity to gauge the success of our methods. In almost all cases, the stretching produced two results: (1) marked decline of electrical activity in the muscle, and (2) partial to complete relief of the pain (see Figure 6-1).

Over these years of experimentation we eventually learned how to induce muscle pain in volunteer subjects. Then, we were able to run controlled experiments in which we made electrical activity measurements before we induced soreness, during the discomfort, and after we relieved it by stretching.

**Figure 6-1 Static stretching exercises were part of the routine performed by research subjects in Dr. deVries' University of Southern California-AOA study at Laguna Hills Leisure World. (Allan D. Walker)**

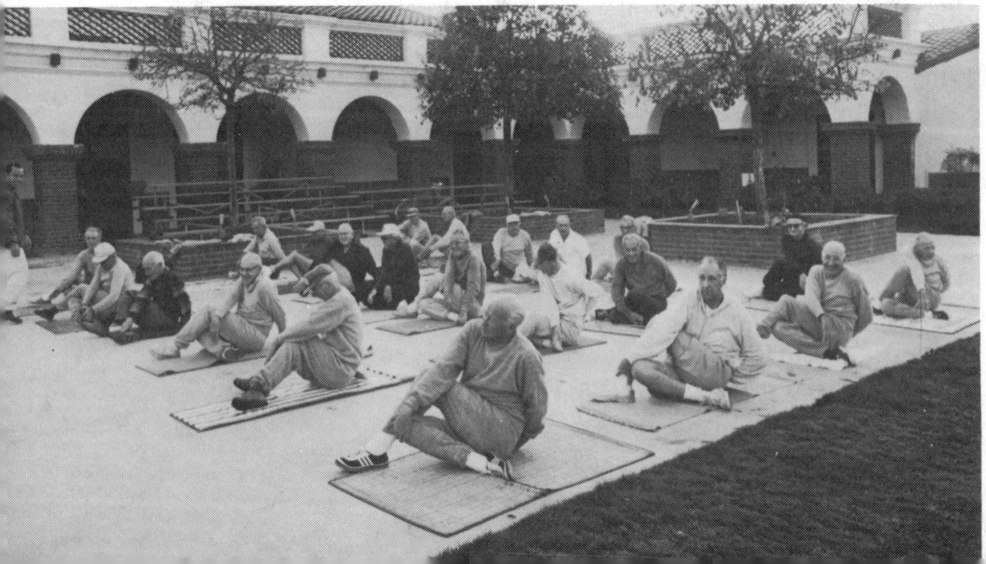

As the result of our experimentation in this area we have formulated a theory which on the basis of known neurophysiological principles further explains the development and continuance of muscle pain when there is no obvious medical explanation such as traumatic injury. I call this the "Spasm Theory" and it goes like this: When a muscle is overworked or *used in a strange position* (which results in overwork for some fibers of the muscle), muscle fatigue ensues. This fatigue in turn results in an inability for the muscle to fully relax (a well-known phenomenon in muscle physiology). Those areas within the muscle which fail to completely relax bring about a local restriction of blood flow because of the increased mechanical pressure upon the small vessels. The relatively inadequate blood flow is called "ischemia." This ischemia is known to result in muscle pain. Now the muscle pain brings about a typical "splinting" reaction involving greater-than-normal muscle activity, in this case contraction, evidenced by a greater number of electrical impulses. The "splinting" reaction is a normal response to immobilize a painful muscle or joint. But it also forms part of the vicious cycle: The original pain causes ischemic pain which in turn causes more local muscle contraction which in turn causes more ischemia which causes more pain, and so on. Thus, we have a very plausible explanation for all the mysterious aches and pains which so often and needlessly (in the absence of injury) accompany the aging process.

To cure this vicious cycle we need to break only one link and the process must run down, with consequent relief of the pain symptoms. The method: stretching the muscles as we described in discussing our experiments.

Again, using the information available in neurophysiology, we find that there are two basic kinds of stretch reflexes in our muscles. The first, called the postural reflex, is a familiar one to all of us.

Physicians commonly test this postural stretch reflex by striking the patient's knee with a small rubber-tipped hammer. The fact that your lower leg swings out shows that the "patellar stretch reflex" is intact. What actually happened is that the blow to your patellar tendon in effect has lengthened (stretched) the quadriceps muscle in your upper leg to which it is attached. The postural reflexes respond to lengthening by automatically contracting—thus, the swing of your leg.

These postural reflexes are set up to maintain the upright position automatically—that is, without any conscious effort on our part. Thus, if we start falling forward (even imperceptibly), the muscles in the backs of our legs are stretched and they respond by shortening to return us to the erect posture before we even know we have deviated from it.

It is important to note that the postural reflex requires little force, but its response is primarily to *quick* stretches. It responds little to very slow stretches.

The second sort of stretch reflex—and the one that concerns us here because of its pain-relieving ability—is the *inverse myotatic reflex* which results from a static stretch. It is quite different from the postural reflex both in its mechanics and its results. It results in relaxation of the muscle instead of a contraction!

Entry into the static stretch is slow and, once entered, the position is held. Thus, the reflex helps to lengthen the muscle rather than fighting lengthening as a jerky stretch does. The static stretch yields muscle relaxation instead of tension. It avoids the postural reflex which would only further aggravate the pain-producing cycle. As we shall see in Chapter 9, the static stretch is used with sufficient force—but *very gently*—to bring about the reflex relaxation to break up the muscle spasm, thus relieving the pain.

We all are familiar with exercise programs that involve bouncing, bobbing, and jerking of muscles to stretch them. You might well ask if my static stretching exercises can bring about the same results. Don't we really have to *force* the muscle into stretching? The answer is no. We have investigated this question and have found that there is no significant difference in the effectiveness of static stretching compared with the jerky sort of stretching exercises.[6] And because the static stretching is much safer for older joints, this is what I have used in all our work with older people. The results have been most gratifying.

### Prevention of Aches and Pains

Ideally, prevention of aches and pains requires the

improvement of several elements of physical fitness, of which joint mobility is probably the most important. In addition to flexibility, we need an optimum level of muscular strength and endurance. This is so because if our muscles are weak and flabby, the smallest physical chore is sufficient to bring about the muscle fatigue which may result in our previously described vicious cycle.

We also need good posture and good movement patterns. If we move in such a way as to place all the strain of even a light load on just a few fibers of a small muscle, the fibers will become overloaded and then fatigued, leading to muscle spasm. Good posture is important because it helps balance all our body segments, and prevents overloading of any one or a few postural muscles. In contrast, poor posture, whether in sitting, walking, or standing, or as required in certain business or professional activities, results in overstretching one set of muscles while others are allowed to shorten.

We have shown that maintaining a muscle in a shortened condition is the best possible way to bring about muscle pain. In fact, this is one of the methods we used to induce muscle spasm for investigation in the laboratory. Thus, the dentist who often must stand for long periods with head, neck, and shoulders cocked at odd angles is particularly prone to back problems.

To understand why poor posture and poor movement patterns can be blamed on muscle structures, it's important to realize that all our joints are surrounded by *pairs* of muscles, each of which can only produce force in shortening. Take the elbow joint for example: When the flexor muscles (biceps, etc.) shorten, they move the hand and wrist closer to the shoulder. Their opposite number, the extensors (triceps, etc.) on the back of the upper arm, have the opposite function. When one of such a pair of muscles shortens at the command of the nervous system, the other must give way or a tug of war would ensue. The nervous system takes care of this by reflexes. These reflexes ordinarily insure that when one muscle is switched on, the other is switched off. But even when it's switched off, a considerable passive resistance remains in a muscle and its associated structures. The resistance grows greater as the muscle is allowed to remain for long periods in a relatively shortened state. It is this increased resistance that causes the restricted movements of older people.

How do we explain the commonly observed stooped posture in the inactive older person? In many cases, we can find our answer in shortened muscles. The poor posture probably is the result of a lifetime in which sedentary habits have almost never required the extension of the cervical (neck) area into its full range. Long hours spent reading, working over a sewing machine, at a desk or workbench, all result in allowing the neck and trunk flexor muscles to remain shortened. Eventually, as we grow older, deposits of calcium salts in the joints themselves might complete the process of immobilization. For persons in which this calcification process has become far advanced, nothing can be done for relief.

But how much improvement can physical conditioning—strengthening and stretching of muscle tissue—provide in reducing joint stiffness in the relatively normal older person? To attack this problem in our laboratory, we had to be able to measure joint stiffness in reasonably controlled experiments. Toward this end, we assembled electronic instrumentation around the basic principles established by Drs. Johns and Wright at Johns Hopkins and by Dr. Charles Long and his group at Case Western Reserve Medical School. Gearing up with the same basic electromyographic technique that we used in the studies of muscle pain, we specifically set out to measure stiffness of finger joints. At the present time only the finger joints can be so measured, because the tissue masses involved with other joints are too large. Previous measurements of finger joints by other scientists have verified the rather obvious fact that older people do have increased levels of stiffness in the finger joints.

Elizabeth Chapman, one of my National Institute of Child Health and Human Development doctoral fellows, chose this area of research for her dissertation at USC's Ethel Percy Andrus Gerontology Center. She examined the effects of a finger exercise program on joint stiffness in 20 young men and 20 older men and found that *significant improvements in joint mobility resulted in both age groups.* Interestingly, *the old improved as much as the young.*[7]

We have since repeated the experiment, using only a general physical conditioning program with no special exercises for the fingers. Again, we saw significant exercise-induced benefits in better finger joint mobility.

It would be most unscientific to draw any final conclusions from two relatively small experiments originating in the same laboratory. But it is safe to say that the data suggest the importance of physical conditioning in maintaining good joint function.

### Summary of Our Evidence About Relieving Joint Stiffness

To summarize, the scientific evidence available at present indicates that:

1) Muscles which are maintained for protracted periods in a shortened state become very difficult to stretch.
2) We require frequent movement activity which stretches all our muscles throughout their full range to maintain sound functional joint structures.
3) In the absence of arthritic damage, at least, exercise which improves the strength of surrounding muscles can result in better joint function.
4) Muscular aches and pains appear to be related in many instances to joint stiffness arising from inactivity and subsequently impaired muscle function.

It appears to me that the best insurance (probably the only insurance) against the aches and pains that so often accompany the aging process (without any underlying disease) is that of maintaining an optimum level of physical fitness with appropriate emphasis on improvement of joint mobility.

Improved joint mobility is very likely to be accompanied by the unexpected dividends of better posture, a springier step, and all the improvements in one's appearance that these imply.

For all of these reasons, we include as part of our exercise program a simple series of static stretching exercises. These are designed to help maintain your joints and muscles in such a state that you will be able to "hang loose," in the vernacular of our younger generation.

# 7

# FAT VS. MUSCLE: A WEIGHTY PROBLEM

## Controlling Your Weight

"Everybody loves a fat man."

"Adolph," the proverbial portly gentleman asks his valet, "are the shoes I have on shined?"

So go the ruminations of the punsters, funsters, and would-be philosophers on the subject of people who are overweight. But from the standpoint of human health, there's nothing really funny about it. There are very few very fat very old people around. The national statistics clearly indicate that longevity *does not mean* survival of the fattest.

Unfortunately, there have been as many pieces of misinformation produced about human overweight as there have been attempts at humor. The result is that many people, duped by unscientific supposition, have misconceptions about overweight and proper ways of reducing. The misconceptions can be downright dangerous, as in the case of the severely obese person who, instead of seeking medical supervision, embarks on a starvation diet or other equally violent regimen. Some advertisers who tout their "sure-fire" weight reduction methods take advantage of people who don't realize the product or system is, in fact, unscientific—based on fad or quackery. Misconceptions also can result in severe discouragement when reducing methods don't seem to be working, even though the person adheres to the regimen religiously. The discouragement in turn frustrates further efforts to reduce. Let's set the record straight by taking a look at the proven physiological principles underlying weight control.

We can begin by saying that exercise plays a significant role in reducing and maintaining proper body weight in persons of any age. This has been proved scientifically over the years in many studies, including our own research into the effects of exercise on older people.

### Two Important Points About Weight Control

Let me emphasize two important points at the outset:

*First:* It is not really *weight loss* we are after; it's *fat loss.* The two are not the same because of the human body's composition. The body is made up of active tissues and inactive tissues. The active tissues comprise muscle, glands, internal organs, and so forth—in short, the protoplasm which is necessary for all our living processes. The inactive tissue is fat. While it's true that we need small amounts of fat to serve as padding for internal organs and as insulation under the skin, the proportion of body fat should not exceed 14 to 15 percent in men and 20 to 22 percent in women.

*Second:* I make no claim for exercise as a panacea for all obese people. In the severely obese, for example, vigorous exercise would be ill-advised until some weight reduction had been brought about by dietary restriction under the direction of a physician. Although exercise can certainly make a contribution, medical supervision is necessary to protect the severely obese person from overstrain, particularly of the cardiovascular system and connective tissues, such as tendons and ligaments. For the moderately overweight individual, however, the best solution is a combination of diet and exercise until normal weight is achieved. Once this is accomplished, normal weight can be maintained with our exercise regimen alone if dietary intake is appropriate for the level of physical activity.

### A Testimonial

One of the more interesting testimonials we received from participants in our USC Administration on Aging study was that from M. R., who at age 67 began our program considerably overweight. Six months later, he had lost 25 pounds. This was not entirely attributable to the exercise program, however, because he also voluntarily restricted his caloric intake, especially the sweets in his diet. What is most interesting here is not the fact that he lost weight. This we have learned to expect. Most intriguing is the contrast between his weight loss in our exercise program with a similar effort some years earlier, when M. R. had undertaken a rigorous diet without exercise. After bringing his weight down to normal, he felt chronically tired—"dragging"—with little or no energy to do much of anything. Out-of-state friends whom he saw only periodically commented on his poor appearance. But years later, after the weight loss of about the same magnitude in our program, using the combination of diet plus exercise, he felt fine and he had large energy reserves. The same friends, on a subsequent revisit, commented on his improved appearance and obvious good health.

Is this an unexplainable or unusual occurrence? Not really. For one part of the answer, it has been demonstrated that about 65 percent of the weight loss in fasting men consists of active tissue (such as muscle) loss. Only 35 percent of it is fat loss.[1] In contrast, physical conditioning brings about small increases in the active tissue mass, while the fat is slowly melted off, if dietary intake of calories remains constant. This fact can help us better understand the problems accompanying M. R.'s earlier weight reduction effort. A loss of vital active tissues is the probable explanation for his "dragging" fatigue; and loss of connective tissues may well have accounted for increase in skin sags and wrinkles which his friends noticed in commenting on his poor appearance. The most likely reason for the favorable result after the diet-exercise regimen is that he was *losing fat*, not muscle and connective tissues.

**Fat-Loss or Weight-Loss?**

We saw the same basic principle at work in our other participants, although most of them didn't lose as much weight as M. R. Remember that our subjects were chosen for their basically good health, and therefore none was seriously overweight. Further, the research did not include a diet component. Nevertheless, our exercising subjects, on a group average, lost a little over 1 percent of their body weight. Most important, they lost 3.6 percent of their body fat. In other words, *they lost over three times more fat than weight.* This demonstrates the beneficial effect of exercise compared with diet alone. With exercise, the person loses the inactive tissue—the inert fat—without losing the vital active tissues.

By now, you may be saying, "Certainly this discussion is

not for me. I still weigh the same as I did when I was in college." Good for you. Then you're really not as badly off as most of your peer group, provided your weight was normal in the college years. However, don't put the book down yet. Perhaps you're not sloppy fat—but if now at age 60 or 70 you're the same weight which was normal for you at age 20, you are between 12 and 15 percent overweight. This is because we lose about 3 percent of our active tissue per decade on the average. In other words, the lost active tissue has been replaced by fat if your weight has remained constant, so you're actually overweight.

To be more accurate, I should say "overfat" instead of "overweight." It's the excess fat that can lead to such diseases as diabetes, high blood pressure, coronary heart disease, gout, and gall bladder problems.

These tragic results of being overfat are well known to many people. But the actual ways people become overfat in the first place are not so well known to the layman. To explain the basic causes, let's start at the beginning. First, we must recognize that the human organism is in effect a "heat exchange engine." As such, it must obey all the physical laws that govern energy exchange. Here's the basic equation explaining net energy exchange and expressing the processes of metabolism:

Calories Taken In
Caloric Balance = (minus)
Calories Expended

We're all aware that different foods have varying caloric content, and that we take in these various amounts of calories in the foods we eat. We expend calories in three basic ways: 1) in basal metabolism, which is the base rate at which we burn energy for survival; 2) in what we call "work metabolism," that is, the increased rate of energy expenditure when we are exercising or involved in any physical activity; 3) finally, some calories are lost from the system in the excreta.

### Calories and Energy

If an individual takes in more calories than he expends, he is in a positive energy balance. He has an energy excess. Now the law of energy conservation tells us, energy can neither be gained nor lost, it can only be changed in form. Therefore, what becomes of this excess energy? It is changed into body fat. An individual would gain approximately one pound of fat for every 3,500 excess calories.

Conversely, if an individual expends more energy than he takes in, a negative caloric balance will result. And he will burn fat (converted energy) in order to make up the deficit. This fat loss occurs at the rate of approximately one pound of fat for

**Figure 7-1**

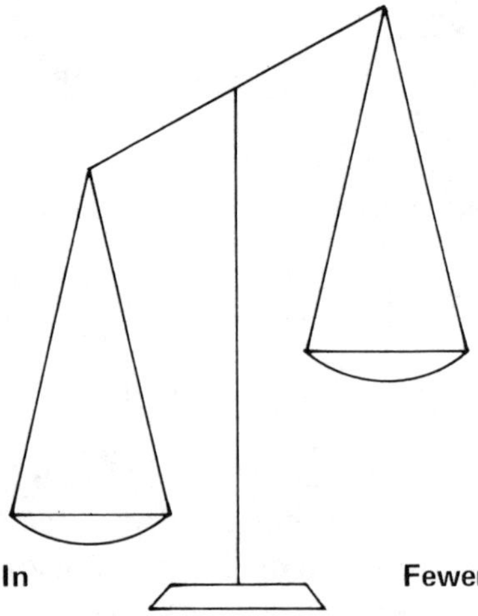


The Positive Energy Balance → Fat Gain

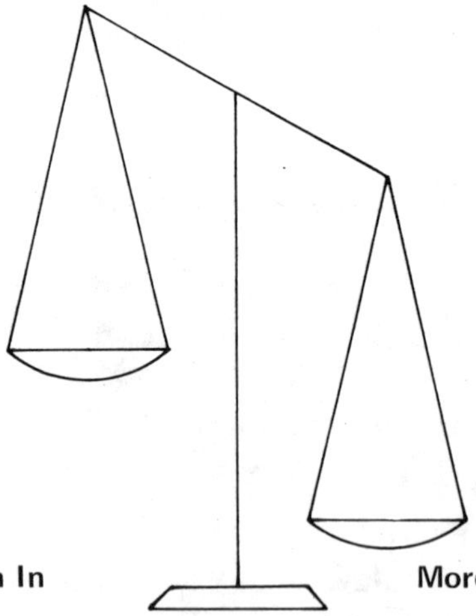


The Negative Energy Balance → Fat Loss

every 3,500 extra calories spent. Therefore a negative caloric balance is what we wish to achieve in order to lose fat. And exercise, which increases energy output, is part of this process.

Figure 7-1 helps us to visualize the basic energy exchange law. At the top, where the scales are tipped to the left by calories taken in—in excess of those expended—we have the positive energy balance. The excess of calories will cause a certain amount of fat to be deposited. At the bottom, however, the scales are tipped to the right, indicating that more calories are being expended than taken in. By keeping in negative energy balance, the fat is melted off slowly but surely.

It is *during* exercise or increased physical activity that the metabolic rate goes up, causing energy (fat) loss. Interestingly, however, it has been known for many years that the resting metabolic rate remains higher than normal for some hours *after* the exercise bout. We investigated this increased metabolic rate further in our laboratory. In a controlled experiment, it was found that the resting metabolic rate was from 7.5 to 28 percent higher four hours after a vigorous workout than at the same time on "nonexercise" control days. The higher rate was shown to persist for at least six hours after exercise. This effect of exercise—over and above the energy cost of the exercise itself—would have resulted in a weight loss of 4 or 5 pounds per year if the individuals tested had exercised daily. Thus, in a sense, exercise keeps working toward your weight reduction goal hours after you sit down to rest.

A most important point here, however, is that the metabolism equation does not dictate the rate at which weight can be gained or lost. Obviously, a pound of weight is lost if we go into a negative caloric balance of 3,500 calories at a rate of 100 calories per day for 35 days or 350 calories for ten days. In the first case, we lose a pound in 35 days, and in the second, one pound in ten days. Many people have been discouraged from using exercise to reduce weight because of misleading "salesmanship" which states the need for 36 hours of walking—or other ridiculously heavy workloads—to lose one pound. It is indeed undesirable, as well as impossible, to try to lose one pound per day in this fashion. However, by applying only a very low level of salesmanship and sound physiology, we might say that walking an extra half hour per day would result in a weight loss of five pounds per year—and it is the "long haul" that counts.

To recapitulate the physiological realities of weight control, we can say from the standpoint of energy metabolism that obesity is necessarily the end result of a positive energy balance. Although this is a great oversimplification, it will aid in understanding the problem. Therefore, only three alternative methods are available for the reduction of weight: (1) increased energy expenditure and constant food intake; (2) decreased food intake and constant energy expenditure; and (3) a combination of methods 1 and 2. The first method can be accomplished by exercise programs; the second by diet. The third, a combination of diet with exercise, is the best method, as we have explained.

### Overweight? The Corrective Prescription Is Exercise and Diet

So, you're overweight, that is, overfat. How do we handle this problem? When obesity gets a start due to inactivity and/or overeating, it is wise to get started with corrective measures as early as possible. The corrective efforts—exercise and diet—should be set up with habit formation in mind. That is, any pattern involving any of the several popular "crash" diets is inadvisable. I say this because when normal weight is regained, a change is necessary, and all too often the change is a reversion to the pre-diet obesity-causing routine. A series of weight gain-and-loss cycles is set up, and discouragement ensues, often resulting in complete loss of control. Severe dietary restriction is a procedure that requires medical supervision. It cannot be treated properly in this book. However, moderate dietary restriction, resulting in weight losses of one or two pounds a week, can be accomplished by estimation of the daily energy expenditure and maintenance of a food intake of 500 to 1,000 calories per day below the caloric energy expenditure level. Information to help you do this is available in various texts on nutrition.

An even more sensible approach would involve a dietary restriction of only 300 to 500 calories per day with a progressive build-up of exercise. An hour a day of vigorous activity would produce another loss of 300 to 600 calories. In this fashion, pleasurable habits can be formed that require no subsequent changes and do not cause the distress of semi-starvation on a crash diet. The reducing process may take a little longer this way, but it will be infinitely more successful.

Although the foregoing basic scientific facts on the use of a combined diet-exercise program for weight reduction are beautifully simple, the actual practice for many millions of Americans is definitely not a simple process once obesity has set in. This is probably due to the interactions of psychological-emotional and social problems with the basic physiology underlying obesity. These are complicated by guesswork and misinformation. As we mentioned previously, we are probably the first culture in the history of civilization for whom major health problems are the result of eating too much and exercising too little. The net result of our modern-day labor-saving devices and our successful avoidance of physical effort—even walking—is predictable. We grow fatter and less fit as we grow older. This aspect of the aging process is totally unnecessary!

A few years back, it was fashionable to place the blame for obesity on endocrine gland malfunctions. This was a popular theory, in that the obese person could handily absolve himself of blame for his overweight. It is true that in a small number of cases, glandular and other malfunctions are the causes of obesity. Medical research, however, has not substantiated the theory for the great majority of overweight people. On the contrary, evidence is accumulating that indicts our sedentary way of life as the real culprit.

Greene, who studied 350 cases of obesity, found inactivity was associated with the onset of overweight in 67.5 percent of the cases, and that a history of increased food intake was found in only 3.2 percent.[2] Pariskova, who analyzed the body composition of 1,460 individuals of all ages, concluded: "One of the most important factors influencing body composition is the intensity of physical activity, and this is true in youth, adulthood, and old age. . . ."[3] Many other scientific investigations, too numerous to cite here, provide indirect support for the belief that lack of physical activity is the most common cause of obesity. Thus, a clear-cut case can be made for the importance of habitual, lifelong, vigorous physical activity as a preventive measure against overweight.

Another misconception is that exercise is not effective in

weight reduction because appetite is automatically increased in direct proportion to the increased physical activity. Mayer and his associates have shown that previously sedentary animals which are given half an hour to an hour of exercise daily actually manifest a *decrease* in appetite.[4] They have shown that this applies to humans as well. It is true that beginning with the second hour of continuous physical exercise, appetite begins to increase proportionately. But that is not what we are advocating in our exercise prescription. We are recommending 30 minutes to an hour daily, the term shown to decrease the appetite.

Women frequently are encouraged to use localized exercises to reduce fatty stores in specific parts of the body, such as the buttocks, hips, and thighs. However, all available evidence seems to indicate that when the negative caloric balance is achieved, the fat comes off in the areas of greatest concentration, regardless of how the exercise is performed. If "spot reducing" has any advantage, it probably is only psychological in nature.

Some interesting new concepts about the physiology of weight reduction deserve comment here. It has been shown that rats trained to eat their entire daily food ration in one to two hours gain more weight than animals that eat whenever they are hungry. It was further demonstrated that the trained rats who concentrated all food consumption into one big meal increased by 25 times the rate at which their fatty tissues incorporated food products into more fat. If these results can be generalized, it would seem that concentrating the greater part of the daily food intake into one large meal has undesirable metabolic consequences—specifically, increase of body fat. Further, skipping breakfast seems undesirable. Indeed, if these data are substantiated by other investigators, a major change in American eating habits is indicated.

Obese people very frequently are discouraged by the results of their dieting. After one, two, or even three weeks of semi-starvation, the scale still may read the same. If they have honestly and strictly adhered to a negative caloric balance, the reason probably is water retention. It has been shown that even though body tissues are being oxidized and the end products excreted, the scale reading may not demonstrate any loss because enough water is retained by the tissues to offset the weight of the oxidized tissues. This water retention cannot continue indefinitely, however, so that the predicted weight change will eventually occur, although it might not follow the day-to-day caloric deficit. Forewarned is forearmed: Don't be discouraged when the desired result is delayed; it may well be attributable to temporary water retention.

It should be emphasized that weight control is best carried out as a matter of habit formation, which automatically takes care of the "long haul." This should include the development of physical skills that will permit, indeed encourage and motivate, regular participation in vigorous activities such as hiking, jogging, swimming, and so on. Such activities are enjoyable and can be performed with a minimum of cooperation by other persons. A person who develops these habits and participates regularly—at least twice, and preferably three or four times a week—will seldom have to be unduly concerned about his diet. With normal moderation in eating, including a gradual decrease in caloric intake with age, in all likelihood he will have no problems with obesity.

As a final note, if you question the effectiveness of exercise for losing weight, you can most readily see the answer not in research, but in the empirical wisdom of mankind's experience. Obesity is practically unknown among the healthiest persons, such as athletes and heavy laborers, many of whom daily consume prodigious amounts of food. By virtue of their lifestyles, they easily maintain the proper fat-muscle balance. For them, physiologically speaking, there are no weighty problems.

# 8

# THE ALL-IMPORTANT "HOW TO"

## *Self-Testing and Self-Monitoring*

I hope that having come this far, you, the reader, have been sold on the "why" of exercising for better health. By spelling out the benefits our older research subjects realized from only three hours a week of planned and controlled exercising, it was my purpose to get you ready, willing, and eager to dump sedentary habits in favor of the health-giving active life—one that promises a renewal of vigor.

### The Three Elements of the Program

The program I have designed for older people comprises three elements:

1) Exercise of the "endurance" type to condition the heart, lungs, and blood vessels and, concomitantly, to induce relaxation. This consists of a carefully planned walking regimen and/or jogging, depending on your fitness level. Jogging means the slowest possible form of running —a "dogtrot," some might call it.

2) Exercise to strengthen the muscles (particularly those important to good posture). This is built around tried-and-true calisthenics movements selected to accomplish the goals of older men and women.

3) Exercise to improve joint mobility which in turn works toward relief and prevention of the aches and pains that so often accompany the aging process. This is comprised of a series of "static stretching" positions—proven to be a safe and effective means of relieving joint stiffness in older people.

These three basic elements of exercise are developed for you in two levels of difficulty. The lower level, for the less well-conditioned individual, is spelled out for you in Chapter 9. This should be the starting point for most people. It will be sufficient for the entire conditioning needs of many in the *upper* age brackets or for those who have minor infirmities. Chapter 10 describes the Level II program designed as a follow-on to the Level I program of Chapter 9 for those who either (1) already enjoy a relatively good level of fitness upon starting this book or (2) have completed Level I and aspire to the ultimate in physical fitness.

### What Shape Are You in Now? The Program of Self-Testing

With this brief introduction of what is in store for you, let's get on with the business of this chapter, which is essentially to find out what shape you are in *now* through self-testing. Then we can direct you to your appropriate starting point. So sit back (for now), relax, and read the important "how to" steps that are essential for maximum safety and benefit in your exercise program.

## FIRST STEP: LEARNING TO TAKE THE HEART RATE

Because the readership of this book is large and very diverse, the first order of business is for you to establish *your* personal capacity for exercise so that you can determine a program which will be well within your capability and yet intensive enough to get results. To do this, *you must take your own heart rate* at frequent intervals as a measure of your response to the various exercises. Taking your own pulse requires only an inexpensive watch. It can be one with a sweep second hand, such as doctors and nurses wear, or a stopwatch. You may already have the former. If not, I suggest that you buy an inexpensive stopwatch, available in department stores and elsewhere nationwide.

In general, the pulse can be found at any point in the body where an artery can be squeezed against a bony surface. Those of you who have had first-aid courses have already learned this in the use of "pressure points" to stop arterial bleeding. The most convenient places to count the pulse during or immediately after exercise are: at the wrist—the radial pulse; in the neck—the carotid pulse; or on the temple—the temporal pulse.

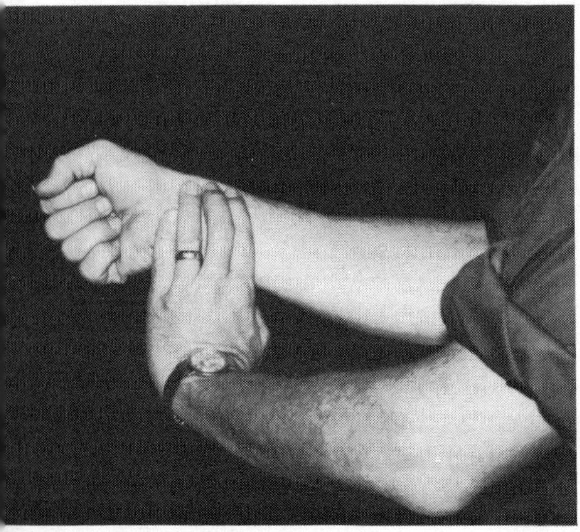

Figure 8-1 Taking the radial pulse.

**1) Taking the radial pulse.** Figure 8-1 shows the location of the radial artery at the wrist. First, locate the large bone of the forearm on the thumb side. This is the radius. Now, moving inward on the palm side of the wrist, you will encounter a rather pronounced tendon. If you will gently place the first three fingers in the hollow between the bone and the tendon, your fingers will rest on the radial artery. Too much pressure will cut off flow entirely and too little will not allow you to feel the pulsation, so experiment to find the appropriate pressure to allow clear and distinct sensing of the pulse. The hand and wrist must be loose and relaxed.

**2) Taking the carotid pulse.** Figure 8-2 shows the location of the carotid artery in the neck. You may use the fingers of the right hand to feel for the artery on the left side of the neck, or, conversely, the fingers of the left hand to locate it on the right side. The artery ascends roughly toward the angle of the jawbone, so placing the pads of the first three fingers gently over the soft tissues of the neck just below the angle of the jaw should put you in contact with the carotid artery. The same instructions given above apply to the pressure to be used in feeling the pulsation. Many people find this artery provides the easiest way of taking the pulse after exercise.

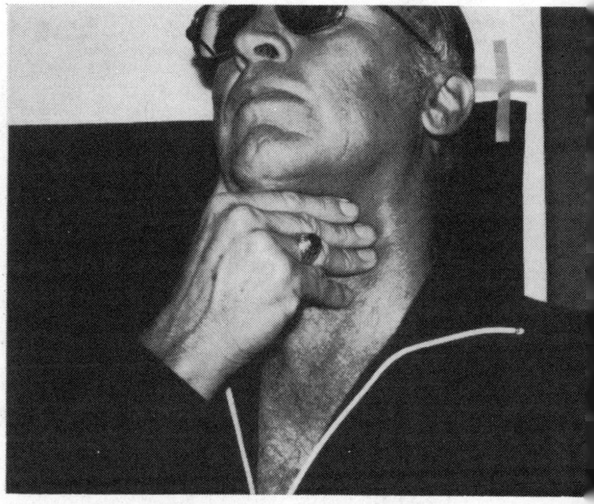

Figure 8-2 Taking the carotid pulse.

3) Taking the temporal pulse. Figure 8-3 shows the location of the temporal artery. Using the same fingers, but this time using the left hand to the left artery or the right hand to the right artery, place the fingers in the wide shallow groove just in front of and slightly above the ear.

Figure 8-3 Taking the temporal pulse.

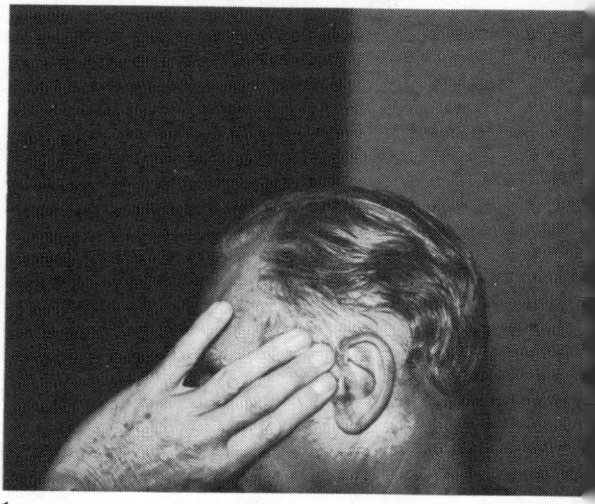

After a period of experimenting you probably will find one of the three arteries more easily than the others. All three arteries will, of course, give you the same information regarding heart rate, so the choice is yours to make.*

Having learned to find the pulse easily and *quickly* at one of the three locations described, you now will practice taking your resting heart rate by one of the two methods described below. If you have a stopwatch, Method 1 is preferable because of the greater accuracy obtained. If you must use a sweep second hand watch, use Method 2.

**Method 1** (for use with stopwatch only)

After finding the artery and establishing the rhythm of your heartbeat, start the stopwatch exactly at a chosen pulse beat which you will count as *"Zero," not "one."* You will then count the following beats as "one—two—three . . . . . twenty." You will stop the watch exactly at the twentieth beat. Now take the time for 20 beats and refer to Table A in the Appendix. From it, you can find the heart rate in beats per minute very easily. For example, if your time for 20 beats was 15.4 seconds, then the heart rate was 78 beats per minute. This method is considerably more accurate than Method 2, but it depends upon precise handling of the stopwatch.

The reason for not counting "one" on the first beat is that the pulse you feel is only one point in a cycle of events which occur with each heartbeat. Thus if you wish to count the last beat as completing the twentieth cycle, then the first cycle must not be counted until its completion, which occurs at the second felt beat. This is really the same idea as calling a baby one-year-old not at birth, but after the completion of one year of life.

The reason for such a short (20 beats) count is that the heartbeat returns to its resting rate very rapidly. Because we are trying to estimate what the heart rate was *during* exercise, the closer in time we are to the actual exercise, the smaller the error.

*For the occasional individual who has great difficulty finding the pulse rapidly, we suggest purchase of an inexpensive stethoscope. The heart sounds can be heard easily if the bell, or diaphragm, is placed 2-3 inches to the left of and below the left nipple.

**Method 2** (for use with a watch with a sweep second hand)

After finding the artery and establishing the rhythm of your heart, start the count with "one" on the first beat after the sweep second hand flies by any major mark on the dial (usually 5—10—15—20 . . . seconds) and end the count on the last beat felt in a ten-second period. If your mental arithmetic is good, multiply by six to get your per-minute heart rate. If you want to do it the easy way, refer to Table B in the Appendix, where the multiplication has been worked out for you.

Practice and test your skill. Having established your method so that you are now able to get accurate repeatable resting heart rates quickly and easily, you are ready for the next test. Climb a moderate flight of stairs and have husband, wife, or friend time you to see how long after reaching the top of the stairs it takes you to find your artery and begin the count. When you can find the artery and begin the count in five seconds or less you are ready for the next step.

I cannot overemphasize the importance of learning to get a reasonably accurate heart rate. Once you have mastered the technique, you can use it to evaluate the stress imposed on your system by any given activity. For example, it would be very sensible to take your heart rate while mowing the lawn in the summer heat or while shoveling snow in the winter, to establish the level of stress involved. Who knows? You might even be able to talk yourself out of the nasty chore! Seriously, the beauty of this simple heart rate measure is that it tells you something about the *total stress* you're under. For example, when mowing the lawn on a hot, humid day, your heart and blood vessels are being stressed not only by the exercise, but also by the heat itself.

Another advantage of this technique lies in the opportunity it affords for better communication with your physician. If you ask your doctor, "Is it safe for me to mow the lawn in the summer?" you have asked a very general question and can expect only an equally vague answer. On the other hand, if you spell it out for him by asking "Is it safe for me to mow the lawn if my heart rate goes up to 165?" then he can give you a specific answer based on what he knows about your physical capacities (or incapacities).

## SECOND STEP: MEDICAL APPROVAL

Now take this book and visit your physician. If you have been religious about your annual or semiannual medical checkups and have had one quite recently, your physician may have enough information about you to advise you over the phone as to your ability to handle a vigorous exercise program. However, if you have been remiss with regard to medical checkups for some time, then you should not be unhappy if your physician insists upon considerable lab work and a lengthy examination, probably including a resting electrocardiogram, at least, and possibly an exercise stress test.

In any event, you must clear the exercise program with your doctor because exercise is like a potent drug—after age 25, it is not for everyone, nor is it to be taken indiscriminately. In the previous chapters I have outlined the many health benefits which improved physical fitness can provide for you. But there also are certain medical conditions in which vigorous exercise might be ill-advised. In such a case only your physician can counsel you.

Point out to your doctor, however, that this exercise program has been professionally designed and is based on many years of research on older people. The results have been published in the medical literature. The prescription is directed specifically to men and women over 50. Consequently, you will be led into the program very gingerly. In fact, you will not engage in exercise that raises your heart rate above 120 throughout Level I. And in Level II the heart rate limit is 140 for the 50- and 60-year-olds and 130 for those over 70.

Many reasonably healthy people over 50 may have physical impairments which, though not life-threatening, may cause concern in the physician's mind regarding involvement in a truly vigorous exercise regimen (such as that in our "advanced" course, or Level II). If this is the case for you, then show him the Level I regimen. This is the starting level for everyone except the well-trained older athlete, and we have shown in our laboratory tests with older people that even this low-level activity can bring about very significant improvement in health and physical fitness. Level I is very similar to Level II with two major differences: The calisthenics are done more slowly in Level I; and Level I involves progressive walking instead of the more vigorous "jog-walk" of Level II. In Level I, you will set the upper limit for your heart rate at 120. Because this is no higher than you often achieve in normal, everyday exercises such as in climbing stairs, the program should be safe for anyone who is ambulatory. However, *the final decision still rests with your doctor.*

Now, having gained your physician's approval, ask him to verify the accuracy of your heart rate monitoring procedure. This is very important because your health and maximal improvement depend upon your working at just the right level. Too little means no improvement; too much also means no improvement—plus possible hazard. While you take your heart rate by the procedure described above, he also will take your heart rate simultaneously. If three consecutive checks under resting condition show no error greater than three beats per minute, you probably are doing an adequate job.

You also should ask him to check your pulse-taking at a higher heart rate, such as that induced by stepping up and down, floor to low stool, or by jumping up and down for about 30 seconds. This will have the added advantage of allowing your doctor to observe your response to exercise. Under these conditions, your count should be within four beats per minute of your doctor's count.

## THIRD STEP: SELF-TESTING

Now you're ready to do the preliminary self-evaluation of your physical fitness. We need this basic information at the start for two reasons: It will help you tailor the program to your personal needs; and it will enable you to measure your own improvement as you progress from step to step in the program. The latter is particularly important to you because there is no better motivation than that of monitoring progressive improvements. You see that it's all worthwhile.

The self-testing, which we call the Progressive Pulse Rate Test, is simple and easy.[1,2] It begins with a very light, slow workload which will not stress the normal older person too severely; consequently, there is little likelihood that sore muscles will result. Done in the privacy of your home, it requires no sophisticated or expensive equipment.

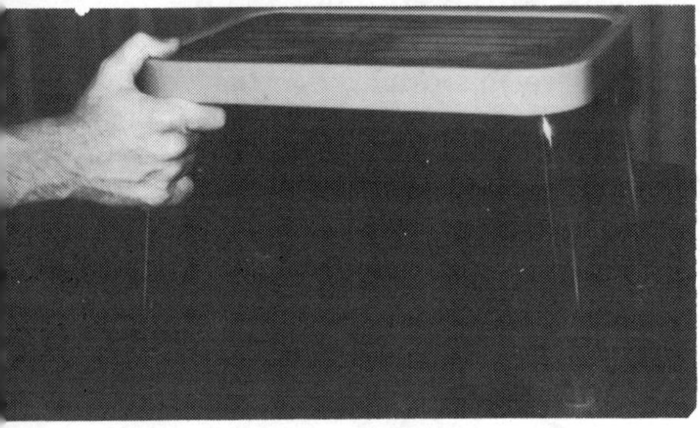

Figure 8-4
A useful kitchen stool for testing.

Here's the equipment you'll need:

• A Sturdy Kitchen Stool—This should be 10 to 12 inches high, with a non-slip surface on top and bottom. You already may have one of these. If not, such stools are available in department and hardware stores at a nominal cost (Figure 8-4).

• Stopwatch or Wristwatch with Sweep Second Hand

• Cadence Counter—this can be a metronome such as is used by musicians for their practice—if there's one available. If you do not have a metronome, you can use a simple pendulum which we will show you how to set up simply and easily. All you need are a 30-inch length of strong string or fish line, several heavy washers, and a thumbtack.

Now, here's a preliminary look at the Progressive Pulse Rate Test:

The entire test consists of stool-stepping. It is done in a four-step cycle. Count "one" as you place your left foot on the stool. Count "two" as you lift your entire body weight onto the stool by placing your right foot alongside the left on the stool. Count "three" as you step down to the floor with the left foot. Count "four" as you bring the right foot back down. These four steps constitute one complete cycle. Figures 8-5 through 8-8 show you the way it looks.

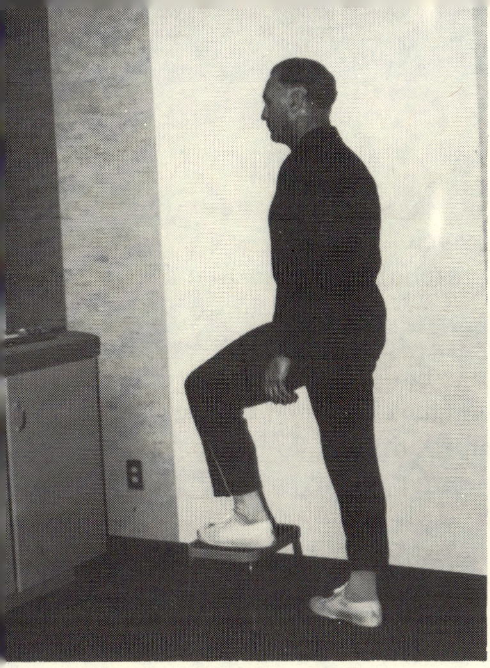
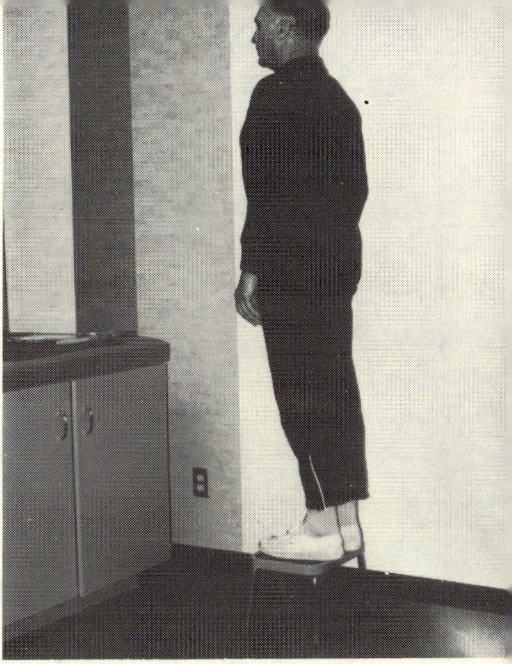

Figure 8-5 Count "one"

Figure 8-6 Count "two"

STOOL-STEPPING

Figure 8-7 Count "three"

Figure 8-8 Count "four"

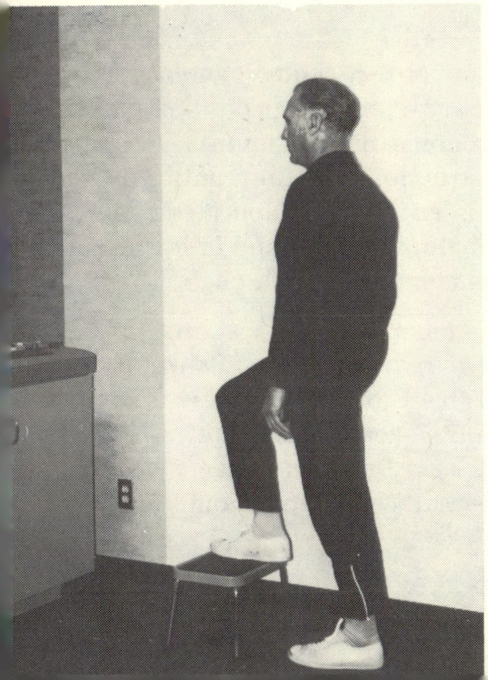
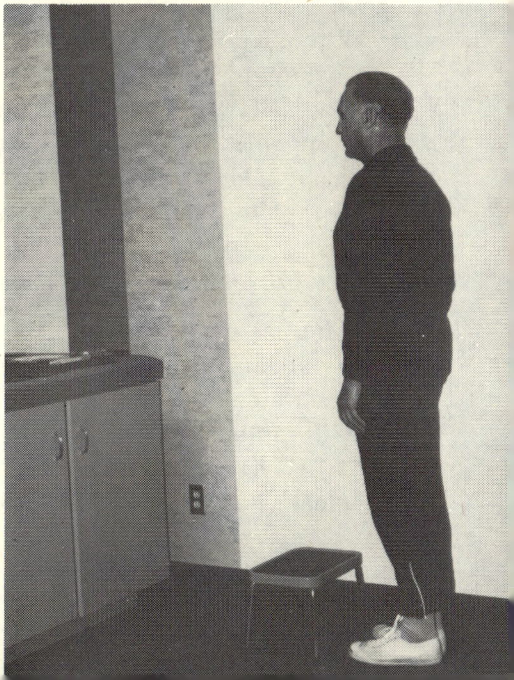

Sound simple and easy? It is.

Now, in order to familiarize yourself with the test, do some slow practice of the four-step cycle.

Be sure that you are fully extending the knee and hip joints as you stand atop the stool. The test is set up to relate your heart rate to a standard stress, which is measured as the height to which you are raising your body weight. If you don't fully straighten up at each step, you haven't raised your weight the full height of the step, and your results will not be accurate.

Is that all there is to it, you ask? Basically, yes. The only additional factors in the actual test are timing each step and count in specific rhythmic cadences (that's what the metronome or pendulum is for), and taking your pulse between bouts of stool-stepping.

The Progressive Pulse Rate Test consists of four one-minute bouts of stool-stepping. In the first minute, you do 12 four-step cycles (48 steps). In the second minute, you do 18 four-step cycles (72 steps); in the third minute, you do 24 four-step cycles (96 steps); in the fourth minute, you do 30 four-step cycles (120 steps).

Between each of these one-minute bouts, there's a rest period.

The best way to approach the test is to practice it, doing a complete run-through one day, and to actually take it for results the second day.

**The First Day**, as we said is for practice. Now is the time to make mistakes and correct your errors. Fully familiarize yourself with the use of the necessary equipment, coordinating step with cadence counter (metronome or pendulum). Don't rush; take your time. Read all instructions carefully until you completely understand. The test is not very complicated; it's just a question of putting all the factors together and following the procedures in sequence. Do one complete run-through.

**The Second Day**, you'll be fully familiar with the test and will be able to proceed with dispatch, assured that the results will be accurate. Record your results in Table C of the Appendix. This will establish your starting point in the exercise program.

The test should be taken at least one hour after a light meal. To make the test a valid measurement, you should have had no coffee, tea, or other stimulants, nor should you have exercised vigorously or smoked for several hours previously. Room temperature should be between 70 and 80 degrees. No binding clothes should be worn.

Remember to maintain your stepping cadence as close to the rhythm of the metronome or the pendulum as possible, because the stress on your system also is dependent on how many times you lift your weight in one minute.

**Assemble the equipment:** kitchen stool, wristwatch with sweep second hand or stopwatch, and metronome *or* string, washers, and thumbtack.

**How the metronome is used:** Settings will be: first minute bout—48 clicks per minute; second minute bout—72 clicks per minute; third minute bout—96 clicks per minute: and fourth minute bout—120 clicks per minute. One step is taken for each click of the metronome. If you don't have a metronome, you'll rely on the pendulum timer.

**How you set up the pendulum:** See Figure 8-9a.

**Figure 8-9a Making your own pendulum for timing the stool-step.**

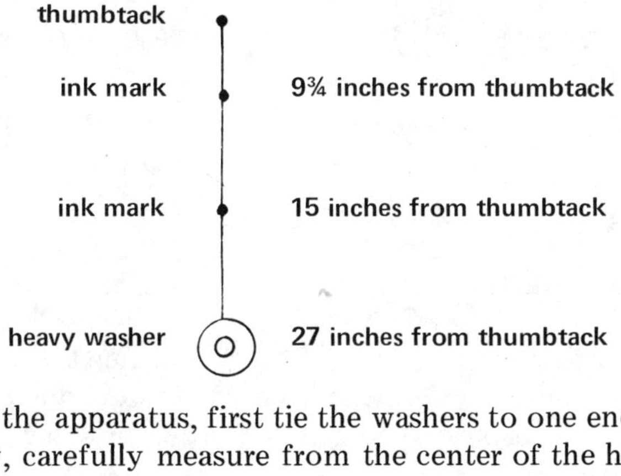


To set up the apparatus, first tie the washers to one end of the string. Now, carefully measure from the center of the holes in the washers (the smaller the holes the better) the following distances down the string, marking each spot with an ink mark: 9 3/4 inches, 15 inches, and 27 inches. These measurements must be accurate. If they are not, the pendulum will not guide the cadence of your stepping accurately. Now, tack the string at its 27-inch mark to the top of a doorway frame, so the pendulum can swing freely a foot in each direction. Set the pendulum in motion, and time the swings for one minute. At 27 inches from center of washer to thumbtack, the pendulum should make 36 complete cycles to and fro. (Another way of saying it is that the pendulum swings to its extremes 72 times per minute; 36 times to the left and 36 times to the right.) Test this by counting the pendulum's swings, using your sweep second hand or stopwatch. The time for 36 complete cycles should be within a second of one minute. If not, you have measured incorrectly.

How the pendulum is used: See Figure 8-9b.

**Figure 8-9b Pendulum method of timing stool-stepping. (The four counts result in one complete stool-step.)**

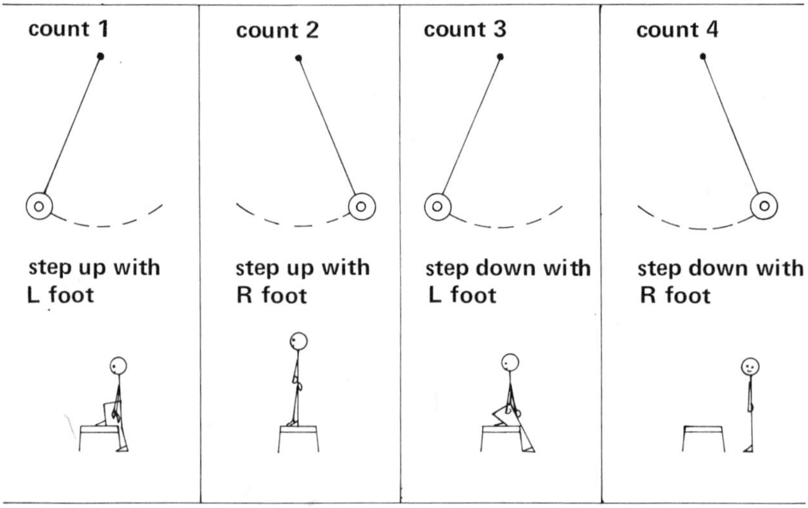


The first step (count "one") putting the left foot onto the stool, coincides with the swing of the pendulum to its extreme left; the second step (count "two") bringing the entire body weight up onto the stool by placing the right foot next to the left, coincides with the next pendulum swing to its right extreme, and so on, as illustrated.

Now, try this. Practice stool-stepping until you have the steps easily coordinated with the pendulum swings over several four-count, four-step cycles. Count "one," "two," "three," "four" aloud at each step.

The pendulum is used only for the 18, 24, and 30 cycle per minute stepping bouts. It is impractical for use with the 12-cycle minute with which you'll be starting, because it swings too slowly at that rate. If you're using the pendulum instead of the metronome, you'll time the first, 12 four-step cycle minute bout by simply doing each four-step cycle in five seconds, as measured by the sweep second hand on the watch. Try this a couple of times to be sure you have the four-step cycle per five seconds mastered.

Now that you've familiarized yourself with the basics of the test and have tried out some of the procedures, you're ready to take the test (Figure 8-10).

## THE PROGRESSIVE PULSE RATE TEST

A. Preliminary

1) Set the kitchen stool about three feet in front of a comfortable chair.

2) Set up the metronome or have the pendulum materials ready.

3) Have a copy of Table C, in the Appendix, and a pen or pencil ready.

4) Hold your watch in your left hand.

B. The First Minute Bout (12 complete four-step cycles)

1) Seat yourself comfortably and count your resting pulse for 30 seconds.

2) After 30 seconds have elapsed since the count, remain seated and count your resting pulse again.

3) If your pulse is stable (plus or minus two beats per minute in the two pulse counts), multiply the 30-second count by two to get

**Figure 8-10 Subject sitting down and counting his pulse after the stool-stepping cycles.**

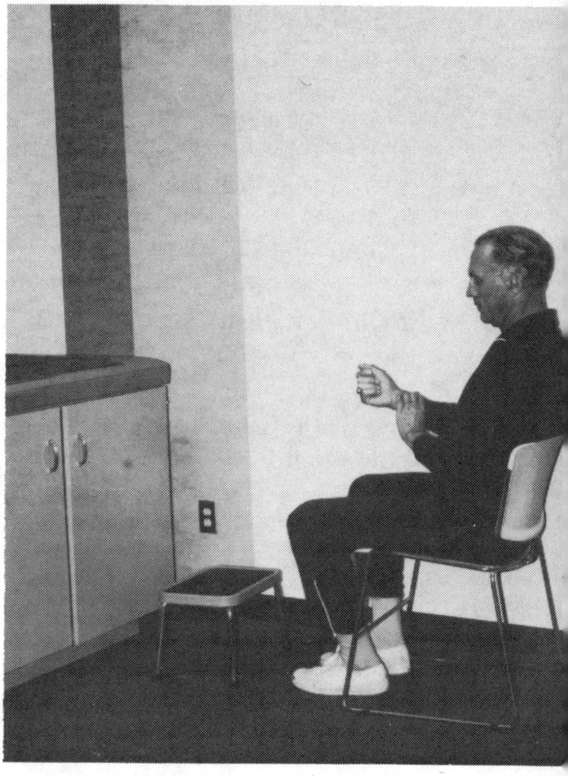

the minute rate. Circle and date the minute rate on Table C and go on with the test. If there is much divergence between the counts, count the sitting pulse again and continue until two successive counts are the same. If after five counts there is still fluctuation, use the average of the five rates for your sitting, resting value and record it.

4) If you are using a metronome, set it to 48 beats per minute, so you will have one click of the metronome for each step of the 12 four-step cycles you will be doing in this first one-minute period. If you don't have a metronome, remember, the pendulum is not used in the 12-cycle bout. In the first minute period, you will be doing each four-step cycle in five seconds, as indicated by your watch.

5) Holding your watch in the left hand, step up with the left foot onto the top of the stool, commencing the first of the 12 four-step cycles. You should take this first step as you start your stopwatch, or as the hand flies by either the "0" or the "30" mark if you're using a wristwatch with a sweep second hand. Aloud, count "one" as the left foot is placed on the stool. Count "two" as you place your right foot alongside the left, lifting your entire body weight onto the stool. Count "three" as you step down with the left foot, and "four" as you bring your right foot back down to the floor. Do 12 complete four-step cycles in one minute. Remember: one step for each click of the metronome *or* one complete four-step cycle each five seconds.

6) As the twelfth four-step cycle is completed at the end of the minute as timed by your watch, seat yourself comfortably in the chair and immediately feel for your pulse.

7) At ten seconds after cessation of stool-stepping, start a *two-minute pulse count.*

8) Record the total count for the two-minute period, not count per minute. Record in the first column of Table C the value that is closest to your two-minute pulse count.

9) Take repeated 30-second pulse counts until your resting rate while seated has recovered to within 10 beats of your original resting value.

### C. The Second Minute Bout

(18 complete four-step cycles)

1) Set the metronome to 72 beats per minute; *or* if you're using the pendulum

method, place the thumbtack through the 27-inch mark (27 inches from center of washer hole to thumbtack) and tack it up where it can swing a foot in either direction. Start the metronome *or* the pendulum swing. Remember, as in the first minute bout, one step and count for each metronome click *or* one step and count each time the pendulum swings to each side.

2) Proceed with steps numbered 5 through 9 in the first minute bout. The only difference between the bouts should be in the cadence and the number of four-step cycles.

**D. The Third Minute Bout** (24 complete four-step cycles)

1) Set the metronome to 96 beats per minute; *or* shorten the pendulum to 15 inches between thumbtack and washer center. Start the metronome *or* the pendulum swing. Remember, as in the previous minutes' bouts, one step and count for each metronom click *or* one step and count each time the pendulum swings to each side.

2) Proceed with steps numbered 5 through 9 in the first minute's bout. Again, the only differences should be in the cadence and in the number of four-step cycles.

**E. The Fourth Minute Bout** (30 complete four-step cycles)

1) Set the metronome to 120 beats per minute; *or* shorten the pendulum to the 9-3/4-inch mark.

2) Proceed as before.

That's it. As you now look over Table C, on which you've recorded your test readings, you have the first indication of your present level of physical fitness. More importantly, you've accumulated the basic data which will tell you at which level to start your exercise program. More about that in Chapter 9.

Looking at your test results, if your score drops by two or more fitness categories as you move to the next higher load, have someone verify your pulse counts on another day. If the same results are obtained then, your exercise results may be abnormal, and the cause for this should be ascertained by a visit to your doctor before continuing with the conditioning program. Figure 8-11 shows the complete record form of a typical, normal response. Figure 8-12 shows an atypical (but not necessarily abnormal) response, in which the heart rate recovery becomes markedly poorer at higher work rates.

**Figure 8-11**

**Scoring Table for Progressive Pulse Rate Test* (Normal Profile)**

| Classification | Total 2 minute pulse count: after 12 4 step cycles per min. | after 18 4 step cycles per min. | after 24 4 step cycles per min. | after 30 4 step cycles per min. |
|---|---|---|---|---|
| | 102 | 110 | 114 | 125 |
| | 106 | 114 | 118 | 130 |
| Excellent | 110 | 118 | 122 | 135 |
| | 114 | 122 | 126 | 140 |
| | 118 | 126 | 130 | 145 |
| | 122 | 130 | 134 | 150 |
| | 126 | 134 | 138 | 155 |
| Above Average | 130 | 138 | 142 | 160 |
| | 134 | 142 | 146 | 165 |
| | 138 | 146 | 150 | 170 |
| | 142 | 150 | 154 | 175 |
| | 146 | 154 | 158 | 180 |
| Average | 150 | 158 | 162 | 185 |
| | 154 | 162 | 166 | 190 |
| | 158 | 166 | 170 | 195 |
| | 162 | 170 | 174 | 200 |
| | 166 | 174 | 178 | 205 |
| Below Average | 170 | 178 | 182 | 210 |
| | 174 | 182 | 186 | 215 |
| | 178 | 186 | 190 | 220 |
| | 182 | 190 | 194 | 225 |
| | 186 | 194 | 198 | 230 |
| Poor | 190 | 198 | 202 | 235 |
| | 194 | 202 | 206 | 240 |
| | 198 | 206 | 210 | 245 |

*H. A. deVries, K. S. Ambe, and G. M. Adams, Unpublished data.

**Figure 8-12**

**Scoring Table for Progressive Pulse Rate Test* (Atypical Profile)**

| Classification | Total 2 minute pulse count | | | |
|---|---|---|---|---|
| | after 12 4 step cycles per min. | after 18 4 step cycles per min. | after 24 4 step cycles per min. | after 30 4 step cycles per min. |
| | 102 | 110 | 114 | 125 |
| | 106 | 114 | 118 | 130 |
| Excellent | 110 | 118 | 122 | 135 |
| | 114 | 122 | 126 | 140 |
| | 118 | 126 | 130 | 145 |
| | 122 | 130 | 134 | 150 |
| | 126 | 134 | 138 | 155 |
| Above Average | 130 | 138 | 142 | 160 |
| | 134 | 142 | 146 | 165 |
| | 138 | 146 | 150 | 170 |
| | 142 | 150 | 154 | 175 |
| | 146 | 154 | 158 | 180 |
| Average | 150 | 158 | 162 | 185 |
| | 154 | 162 | 166 | 190 |
| | 158 | 166 | 170 | 195 |
| | 162 | 170 | 174 | 200 |
| | 166 | 174 | 178 | 205 |
| Below Average | 170 | 178 | 182 | 210 |
| | 174 | 182 | 186 | 215 |
| | 178 | 186 | 190 | 220 |
| | 182 | 190 | 194 | 225 |
| | 186 | 194 | 198 | 230 |
| Poor | 190 | 198 | 202 | 235 |
| | 194 | 202 | 206 | 240 |
| | 198 | 206 | 210 | 245 |

*H. A. deVries, K. S. Ambe, and G. M. Adams, Unpublished data.

## FOURTH STEP: FAMILIARIZATION WITH FORMS FOR RECORD-KEEPING

Now is the time to familiarize yourself with the forms provided for your record-keeping. They are found in the Appendix in the back of the book. It is suggested that the reader type or otherwise make his own copies of Tables C, D, and E after the supply provided has been used. Several blank pages follow the Appendix for your convenience.

Table C of the Appendix—pertaining to your self-testing—has been used already. To observe your progress you will retest yourself at 6, 12, and 24 weeks after beginning the exercise program, and at six-month intervals thereafter.

Table D, the daily record form for the progressive walking program, Level I, covers a six-week period.

After a year, the daily record-keeping becomes less important, and daily records can be eliminated unless your doctor would like to see them on the occasion of your regular physical examination. However, it is important to continue to monitor your progress by the PPR Test at least every six months, and the results should be kept and furnished to your physician at each routine checkup.

## FIFTH STEP: WHEN? WHERE? EQUIPMENT NEEDED?

The first question is, "What is the best time to exercise?" Physiologically, I could present arguments for both early morning and late afternoon. I would rule out midday because of the undesirable heat during the summer months. Speaking in the most practical sense, and taking into consideration the strong tendency for most of us to procrastinate and rationalize, I strongly suggest that your exercise period should be first thing in the morning. I suggest you eat a light breakfast early enough so you will have time to do your exercise between breakfast and your normal day's activity.

A related question is "How often?" Our laboratory work was based on three workouts per week. It may be possible to increase the rate of improvement by upping this to four or five per week, but the additional improvement would not be great. In any event, I recommend a minimum of three workouts per week and a maximum of five per week. It is equally important that you do not overwork, because your "batteries need time for recharging."

Where should you work out? The calisthenics and stretching exercises are best done in your bedroom. The progressive walking and the jog-walk are best done in pleasant, hygienic surroundings. Those of you who are fortunate enough to be close to parks, beaches, or other scenic recreational areas should take advantage of them for this part of your exercise program. Running tracks or open roads are equally serviceable, although possibly not so stimulating from the aesthetic viewpoint. City dwellers will need to find a suitable nearby park or schoolyard unless they are able and willing to walk or jog on the city sidewalks.

As to weather conditions, common sense must be applied. The progressive walking program can be continued in all but seriously inclement weather if appropriate clothing is worn. In light rain or snow, or in *moderately* cold weather, you will find your workout particularly invigorating.

"What to wear?" is the next question. Basically, the clothing must be loose enough to allow free movement in comfort. For the calisthenics and stretching exercises in the privacy of your home, loose-fitting casual clothing or undergarments are adequate. For the progressive walking of Level I and the jog-walk of Level II, you will need two layers of clothing, in order that the outer layer can be peeled off as you begin to warm up and sweat. The outer layer should be replaced when cooling down. This is important at the end of a workout to prevent chilling. Make no mistake about it; for the exercise to be beneficial, you will need to sweat. Men tend to perspire more freely than women. But in any event, "sweat" is not a dirty word in our program. I recommend as the basic attire, in order of preference: a warmup suit, a sweatsuit, or light, loose-fitting casual or work clothes. In the summer months, a blouse or T-shirt and walking shorts can be worn under the basic attire. In the winter you will need outer garments, such as a jacket, coat, or sweater, over the basic workout attire, depending on the weather you encounter.

Shoes are very important. For the progressive walking, you should wear sturdy walking shoes, with flat heels and, preferably, with sturdy but flexible rubber soles. For the jog-walk, you must wear either tennis or jogging shoes of good quality. In any event, proper fit is important to prevent blisters.

### SIXTH STEP: MEASURING THE COURSE

Both in the progressive walking and in the later part of the jog-walk program, you will be using distance as one way of making your program progressive. Consequently, you will need a measured distance to traverse. This is most easily gotten by measuring the distance with your automobile odometer, if possible. If you will be using a running track, this type of course is usually one-quarter mile per lap (complete circuit); but in order to be certain it would be wise to determine the length from someone in authority. If you plan to use a footpath or other area in which automobile odometer measurement is difficult or impossible, then I suggest the following procedure: 1) Measure off a half-mile stretch on a road which has an adjacent sidewalk. 2) Walk this half mile, and count the number of paces (one pace is two steps, or each time the left foot strikes). 3) Divide the result by two to get the number of paces per quarter mile.

Now that you've completed these important preparations, the time has come for you to step into a new, more vigorous life with our program of controlled exercise.

# 9

# EXERCISE PRESCRIPTION

## Level I

Now that you're ready for the first day's exercise, the first decision to be made is the starting point—Level I or Level II. So let's look at your scores on the Progressive Pulse Rate Test (PPR Test).

If you were "above average" on all four stepping rates, you are ready for Level II, outlined in the following chapter. However, you must read this chapter first, because the calisthenics and stretching exercises for both levels are described here. After going over each of these and learning them, you can then move on to Chapter 10 for the Level II program.

If you scored in the average or below average categories, you will start here with Level I. Remember, the higher you placed on the PPR Test, the faster will be your progress in the program. In general, you will progress at your own rate, dictated by the extent that your heart rate response to exercise improves. If your physician has reservations about your full participation, you should remain on Level I.

Please remember that every aspect of this program has been developed scientifically in our laboratory. You will achieve the best possible results if you follow the instructions faithfully. I will discuss the reasons for all procedures as we move through the program.

Every workout consists of three phases, *in this order:*

**1) Progressive walking for Level I; the jog-walk for Level II.**

**2) Calisthenics.**

**3) Static stretching.**

The order of these three phases is important because the progressive walking or the jog-walk furnishes an almost ideal gradual warm-up effect, preceding the calisthenics. The calisthenics must be followed by the static stretching in order to prevent muscle soreness which might otherwise ensue in unconditioned older people. This soreness-prevention effect has been studied in our laboratory, and the results have been published in the literature.[1,2]

## FIRST PHASE—PROGRESSIVE WALKING

The first day you will take a leisurely walk for one mile on your measured course. You will want to walk only half the mile "out," leaving the last half for the way back. If you are in very poor condition, you may wish to shorten even this light load. You should complete the mile walk in 20 minutes. At first, however, you will not have developed a "pace sense," that is, the ability to pace yourself, coordinating steps to time and distance requirements. To achieve this you should mark the quarter-mile points as you repeat the exercise on subsequent days. In this way, you can note how close you are to the planned pace, (initially five minutes per quarter-mile). Take your heart rate at the halfway point by the methods described in Chapter 8. Throughout Level I, you will adapt your program in all phases to limit your observed rate to 120 per minute. This will keep the actual "during exercise" rate below 130. Any time you find that your heart rate is above this, slow down the rate of activity, in this case, walking. Record your heart rate on your copy of Table D (see the Appendix). For your convenience, use a small clipboard.

Table 9-1 outlines your progressive walking objectives. The distances and times are approximations. Remember, these should be adjusted if need be, according to your heart rate response.

TABLE 9-1: PROGRESSIVE WALKING OBJECTIVES

| Workout Day | Distance | Time | |
|---|---|---|---|
| 1 | one mile | 20 minutes | 20 min. per mile |
| 2 | 1 1/4 | 25 | |
| 3 | 1 1/2 | 30 | |
| 4 | 1 3/4 | 35 | |
| 5 | 2 | 40 | |
| 6 | 2 1/4 | 45 | |
| 7 | 2 1/2 | 50 | |
| 8 | 2 3/4 | 55 | |
| 9 | 3 | 60 | |
| 10 | 2 miles | 32 minutes | 16 min. per mile |
| 11 | 2 1/4 | 36 | |
| 12 | 2 1/2 | 40 | |
| 13 | 2 3/4 | 44 | |
| 14 | 3 | 48 | |
| 15 | 3 1/4 | 52 | |
| 16 | 3 1/2 | 56 | |
| 17 | 3 3/4 | 60 | |
| 18 | 4 | 64 | |

The table is self-explanatory. If the first-day objective was completed in the time called for (20 minutes), then, on the next workout day, you will do the second-day workout, that is, 1¼ miles in 25 minutes, and so on. If, however, on the first day you either could not complete the distance, or your heart rate exceeded the limit value of 120, then you will continue toward the first-day objective in subsequent workouts until it is completed successfully. This applies to every day's objective. Do not attempt to move on to succeeding objectives until you have achieved all the previous ones.

You will note that the major method of progression employed here is that of increasing distance by modest amounts. This method is used because increasing the distance makes only very small increases in demand on your heart. In contrast, increasing the intensity (speed or rate of walking) necessitates a relatively large acceleration of heart function. The "break" in the table, as you'll note, does not occur until the tenth workout day. That is, the intensity (speed of walking) is not increased until you have completed three miles at 20 minutes per mile. This is called the "double progressive" method, because both duration and intensity are modified.

You should be attentive to your heart rate and achievement of the objective, but keep in mind, *the progressive walking can and should be enjoyable.* Look around. Enjoy the scenery. Whistle, hum, sing, as the spirit moves you. Swing out with an easy gait, head and chest high with a loose, relaxed swing of the arms. By the very act of progressive walking, you are stepping into a new life of improved fitness and vigor!

It is strongly urged that you find a reasonably level area for the walking if at all possible. If only hilly terrain is available then you must be aware of the fact that walking up even a small grade can raise the intensity of the effort required by severalfold. Under these conditions you will not be able to adhere to the schedule shown in Table 9-1. You will then need to be guided entirely by your heart rate. When walking uphill, you will take your heart rate at 30 second intervals and take a 30 second rest whenever it reaches 120 beats per minute. Conversely, walking downhill is less demanding unless the hill is very steep in which case your muscles are working additionally to provide braking action.

One good way to proceed in a hilly area would be to go downhill first (easy warm-up), then come back uphill to the starting point. If the hill is at all steep, I would recommend setting a comfortable distance (one-half to one mile depending upon steepness). Then without modifying the distance as we do on a level course, the progression would be accomplished through decreasing the number of rest periods on the uphill climb. When the climb can be made without needing to stop for rest (heart rate never exceeding 120), your fitness has improved sufficiently to increase the rate at which you have been walking. When the given distance can be negotiated at the most rapid walking rate comfortable for you, then you may elect to increase the distance you walk uphill. Remember, you "mountain climbers" will make just as good progress as the "flatlanders" but you will need to exert more caution and good sense. In fact, if you have been climbing this "mountain" for some period of time, you are probably already in good shape and the PPR test has already referred you on to Level II.

**Benefits:** It is this phase of your exercise program which provides the benefits to heart, lungs, and blood vessels, in addition to the tranquilizer effect, which I have verified in the laboratory, and outlined for you earlier. The progressive walking also demands considerable energy consumption. Consequently, it contributes to weight control.

## SECOND PHASE–CALISTHENICS

As soon as the progressive walking is completed, and before showering, you begin the second phase, calisthenics.

In general, the benefits to be derived from the four simple calisthenics exercises in our program are improvement in muscular strength, endurance, and flexibility.

Table 9-2 gives you a preview of the calisthenics, and the very slow cadences with which you start on the first day.

**TABLE 9-2: PREVIEW OF CALISTHENICS**

| Exercises | Rate | Time | Repetitions |
|---|---|---|---|
| 1) The Bender | 4 per minute | 2 min. | 8 |
| 2) The Easy Push-up | 5 | 2 | 10 |
| 3) Slow-Motion Flutter Kick | 8 | 2 | 16 |
| 4) The Easy Sit-up | 8 | 2 | 16 |

As in the progressive walking phase, your heart rate is the governing factor in progressing to increasing workloads. Accordingly, immediately after completing Exercise 4 of the calisthenics, "the easy sit-up," you must take your heart rate. *Remember:* Your heart rate should not exceed 120 beats per minute.

If your heart rate is below 120, you are free to increase the number of repetitions of the calisthenics on succeeding workout days as far as your heart and circulatory system are concerned. However, *do not increase the number of repetitions to the point of straining or undue fatigue!* There is no need to carry on the exercises beyond about two minutes each. Improvement is achieved by the gradual progression of doing increasingly more repetitions in the two-minute period.

The calisthenics exercises should be done slowly, avoiding all jerky movements. Do not try to force the body further than it will go easily. It is also important that you do not strain on this muscular effort. You can assure yourself of avoiding the straining type of movement by maintaining your normal breathing throughout. If you find yourself needing to hold your breath (particularly on the push-ups), you are working too hard. Straining in calisthenics exercises which results in breath-holding can cause very marked and undesirable increases in blood pressure.

The calisthenics and the upcoming third phase, static stretching, are to be done indoors. Your bedroom might be the best place, because little space is required. You will need only sufficient unobstructed floor space to be able to lie down with your arms outstretched either above the head or sideward.

If the floor is carpeted, you need only provide a large bath towel for cleanliness, to give you a suitable surface for the exercises that involve lying on the floor. If the floor is not carpeted, I suggest using either a straw beach mat or a very heavy beach towel to give you a little cushioning effect. Too much cushioning is undesirable.

Now you're ready to begin the calisthenics. The first time around, you'll want to read carefully and coordinate the instructions with the illustrations of the exercises, to make certain you understand the movements. Then, refer to Table 9-2 for the starting number of repetitions, and begin. Remember to take your heart rate at the conclusion of the fourth exercise.

### EXERCISE 1: THE BENDER

This is a four-count exercise, as shown in Figure 9-1. Starting position is standing with feet shoulder-width apart, hands on hips.

**Count 1:** Bend forward gently but firmly and attempt to touch the floor with your fingers between your feet, *but move slowly; do not force* your hands to the floor.

**Count 2:** Return slowly to the starting position.

**Count 3:** Stretch arms overhead and bend backward as far as you can *easily* arch your back.

**Count 4:** Return to starting position.

**Benefits:** On the way down, the Bender stretches the muscles and connective tissue of the upper back, lower back, and hamstring muscles. On count three, the muscles and connective tissues of the abdominal wall are stretched.

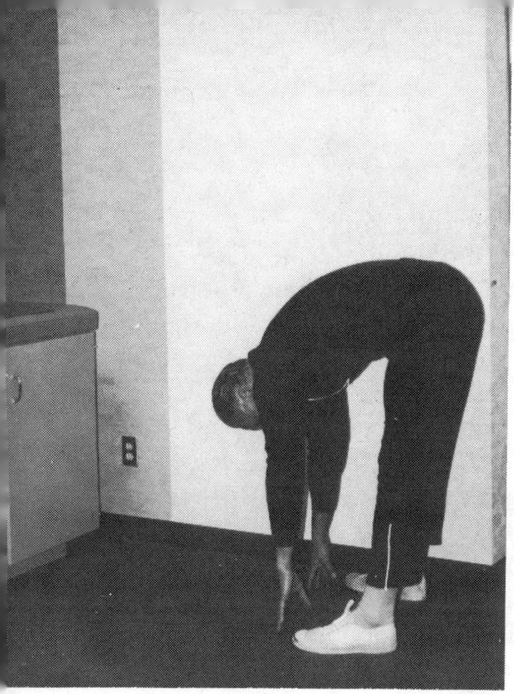

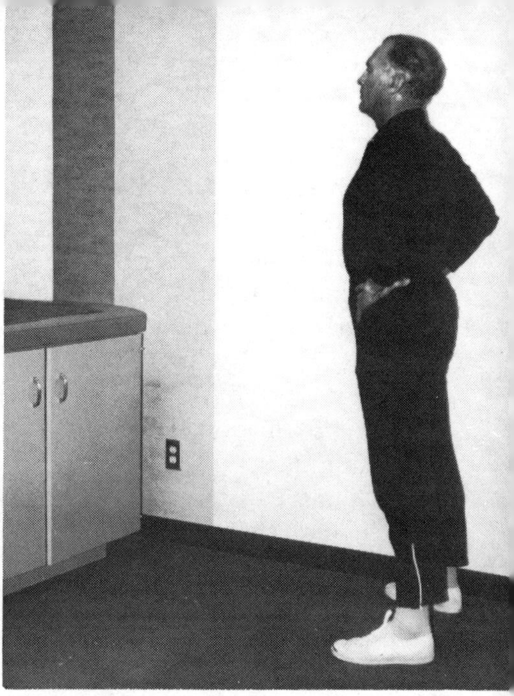

Count 1 Count 2

Figure 9-1 THE BENDER

Count 3 Count 4

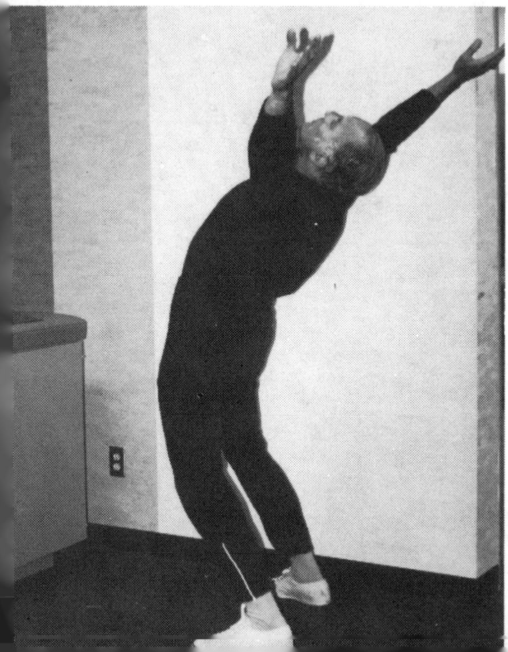

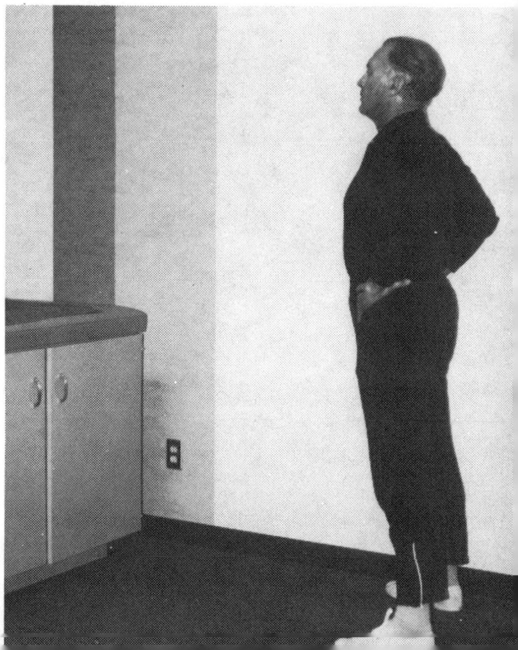

## EXERCISE 2: THE EASY PUSH-UP

This is a two-count exercise, as shown in Figure 9-2. The counting is most easily done as follows: "one-down, two-down,. . ." The starting position is flat on the abdomen with hands alongside the shoulders.

**Count 1:** Straighten the arms, lifting the upper body but leaving the knees and the lower legs on the floor. The body should be straight from head to knees.

**Count 2:** Lower the body gently back to the floor.

**Note:** *Keep the breath flowing* throughout the exercise. Inhale on the upward movement and exhale on the downward.

**Benefits:** Well known in its unmodified form, the Easy Push-up strengthens the muscles of the arms, chest, shoulders, and back. This is important because very few of us do any significant amount of work with those muscles nowadays. It is important that on Level I, the exercise be done in its modified form, as shown in the illustration. In your initial effort you must avoid overstressing and straining. So make it easy on yourself and on your heart by sticking to the Easy Push-Up while you are on Level I of our program. The ladies will not go beyond the "Easy Push-Up" in any event.

**Figure 9-2 THE EASY PUSH-UP**

**Count 1** **Count 2**

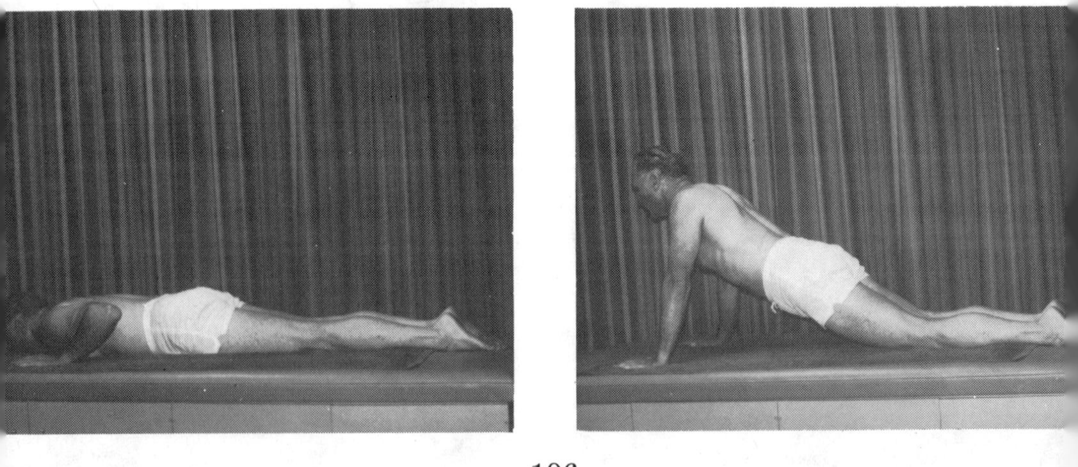

## EXERCISE 3: THE SLOW-MOTION FLUTTER KICK

This is a four-count exercise, as shown in Figure 9-3. Starting position is flat on the belly with hands (palms up) under thighs.

**Count 1:** Lift the head and left leg simultaneously as far as you can *easily*. Keep the leg as straight as possible.

**Count 2:** Return to starting position.

**Count 3:** Repeat with right leg.

**Count 4:** Return to starting position.

**Benefits:** The Slow-Motion Flutter Kick improves function of the very important muscles of the buttocks and low back, as well as the hip extensor muscles, which are critical in the prevention of back problems. Maintenance of good muscle tone is an important goal. So also is an appropriate balance of muscular strength between the front and back of the body. This is one of the sound approaches we can take in the prevention and/or relief of low back pain of muscular origin that troubles so many older people. Our entire thrust with this very brief calisthenics phase is to provide good muscle tone, strength, and endurance for the postural muscles, so your posture and gait will be improved, while the likelihood of your having low back problems is decreased.

Figure 9-3 THE SLOW-MOTION FLUTTER KICK

Count 1

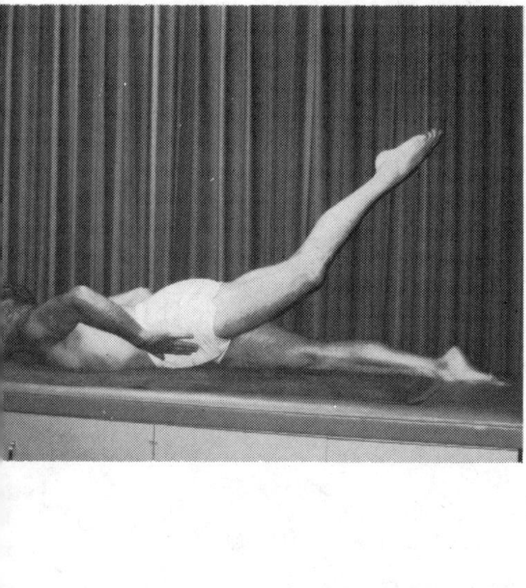

Count 2

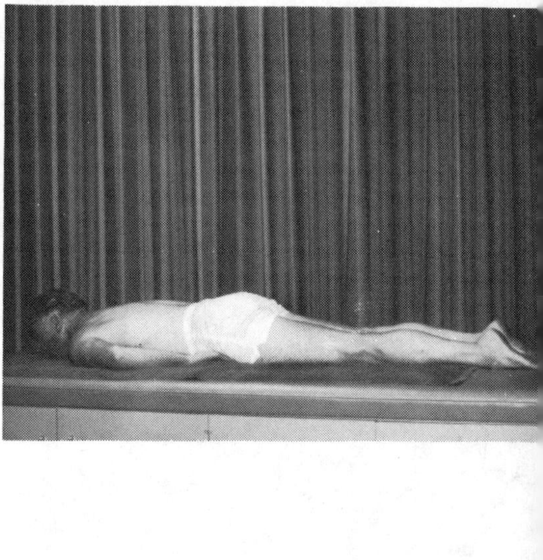

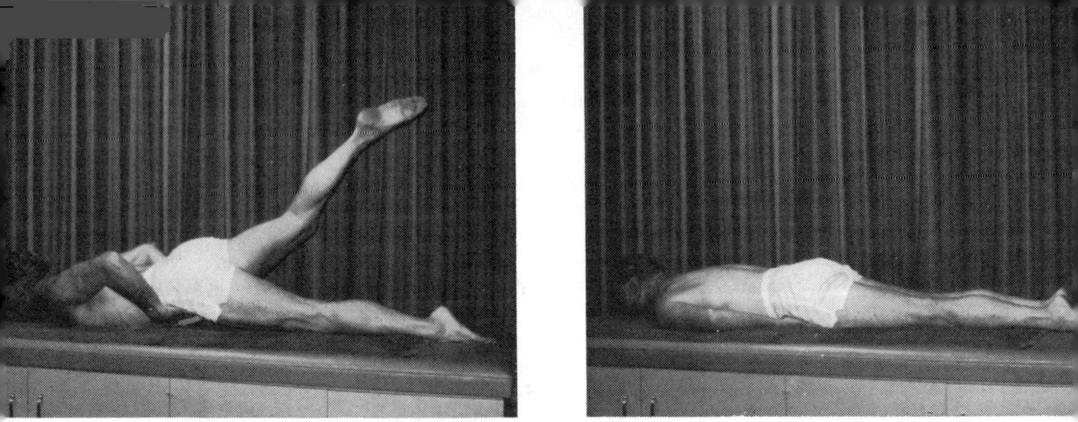

Count 3 Count 4

THE SLOW-MOTION FLUTTER KICK

## EXERCISE 4: THE EASY SIT-UP

This is a two-count exercise, as shown in Figure 9-4. Starting position is flat on the back with hands under small of back, palms down.

**Count 1:** Lift head, shoulders, and upper back (as far as the hands) off the floor by tightening the abdominal muscles.

**Count 2:** Return to starting position. (The starting cadence will probably seem slow to you.)

**Note:** Take heart rate immediately after the last exercise.

**Benefits:** The Easy Sit-Up improves muscle tone in the abdominal wall. This is important to good posture, and may help in relief of low back pain of muscular origin. Do not, however, expect this exercise to remove a "pot belly." Only dietary restriction combined with vigorous activity which burns calories will do that. The first phase of your program, progressive walking of Level I or jog-walk of Level II, is effective in this regard because either activity creates a significant energy demand.

Figure 9-4 THE EASY SIT-UP

Count 1 Count 2

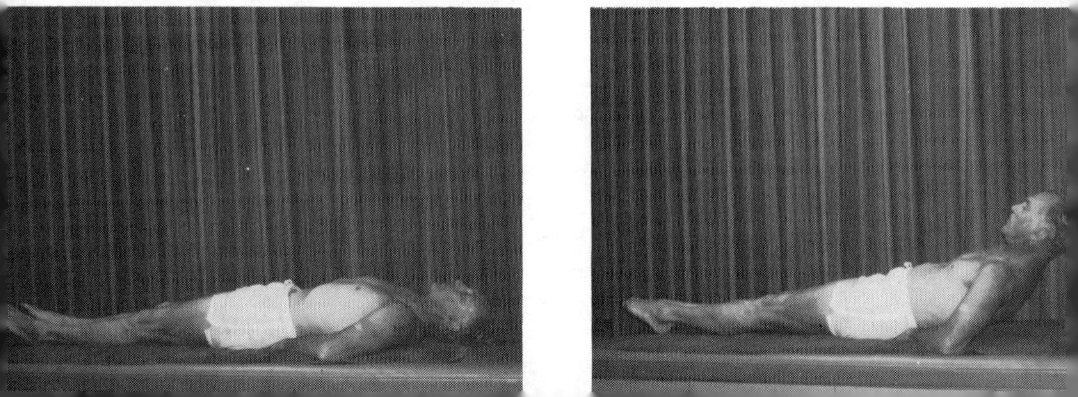

## THIRD PHASE—STATIC STRETCHING

Immediately upon completing the second phase, calisthenics, you will wind up your day's workout with the series of nine static stretching exercises outlined in the forthcoming section of this chapter.

These exercises have their effects through the same basic neurophysiological principles as do the asanas (positions) of yoga. Only recently, scientific research has demonstrated the benefits. Indeed, some of the static stretching exercises are classic yogic positions (asanas). Others are of my own design. The sum total is geared toward accomplishment of our basic aims: prevention of sore muscles and relief of chronic aches and pains; improvement of joint mobility through the safest possible sort of stretching; and aid in bringing about a high level of relaxation after your exercise bout.

I have designed this phase to cover all the muscles and joints you possibly could have used in the first and second phases. Yet the calisthenics and stretching exercises, combined, can be completed in less than 20 minutes after you have mastered the techniques.

Each static stretching exercise is illustrated and described in several different levels of increasing difficulty. It is not expected that many of you will be able to achieve the most advanced level of each exercise the first day. In fact, progress from each intermediate step to more advanced levels might take weeks or months. Continue doing only one intermediate step per day until you can comfortably move on to the next. Remember that the most advanced levels represent your *ultimate goal.* You will work toward it in small easy steps. You might not be able to observe steady progress from day to day. This is not to be expected. But over a longer period of time, the improvement will be realized. How long will it take? The answer depends entirely on you. If you have become thoroughly stiffened up over many years of inactivity, it will take considerable time—possibly a year or longer—to achieve the final goal. If you are overweight, you will find that the extra pounds of fat will "get in your way" and slow your progress.

If you have a history of any serious orthopedic problems, it is in your best interest to take this book and discuss the calisthenics and static stretching exercises with your physician.

There may be an occasional exercise that he would prefer you to skip, even though the entire program has been designed for safe use by older people.

While I advise against performing the first and second phases of the program more than five times per week, the static stretching can be done to good advantage as often as three times a day every day if time permits. This is so because the static stretching constitutes only a very small drain on your energy resources. You always will be working toward the day when you can hold the final position of each exercise for one minute. Progress with the static stretching exercises will be much more rapid if they are done more frequently, although three times a week is sufficient for a slow rate of progress.

When you do the static stretching exercises several times a day, you soon will notice that your flexibility improves as the day goes on, being least in the early morning and best in the evening. This is a normal phenomenon, probably the result of a progressive loosening up of muscles and connective tissues through use during the day and a tightening up due to disuse during sleep at night.

Let me stress that the following static stretching exercises must be performed easily and gently. As in the calisthenics, there is no place for any jerky, bouncing, or sudden movements. Such movements invite nervous reflexes that are self-defeating to our purposes. Do not hold your breath at any time during the static stretching exercises. It is important that you breathe normally.

Indeed, when they are performed easily and in the proper manner, the static stretching exercises will provide an ideal "cooling down" from the more vigorous exercises of the first and second phases. The third phase, static stretching, will leave you in an appropriately *invigorated* but *relaxed* condition.

## EXERCISE 1: THE UPPER TRUNK STRETCHER (FRONT)

Figure 9-5b shows the final position to work toward. Figure 9-5a shows one intermediate step. This should provide enough progression since the Upper Trunk Stretcher is not a difficult position to achieve.

1) Lie flat on the belly, legs straight, toes pointed, fore-

head on the floor, with hands placed palms down under the shoulders.

**2)** Starting with the head and neck, arch upward and backward, inhaling as you go upward.

**3)** Arch the back gradually from the head and neck down as far as the hips.

**4)** Try to achieve as much curvature in the back as possible while keeping the hips and legs flat on the floor.

**5)** Straighten the arms until they are locked.

**6)** Hold the position for 10-15 seconds the first day and gradually, over several weeks or months, increase to one minute. Let down very slowly and easily!

**Intermediate Step**

To make the position easier to attain, three modifications are possible, as shown in Figure 9-5a.

**1)** Place the hands several inches in front of the shoulders to start.

**2)** Leave the legs slightly apart.

**3)** Stop short of full elbow extension in arching the back.

**Benefits:** This position stretches all the muscles of the upper and front part of the trunk, including the abdominal and neck muscles. It also strengthens the muscles of the back which extend the spine. In this way, it helps to improve posture while also helping to prevent low back pain of muscular origin.

**THE UPPER TRUNK STRETCHER (Front)**

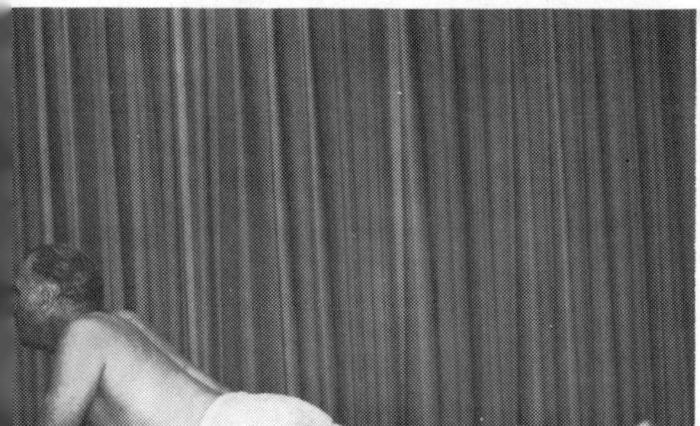

**Figure 9-5a Intermediate position**

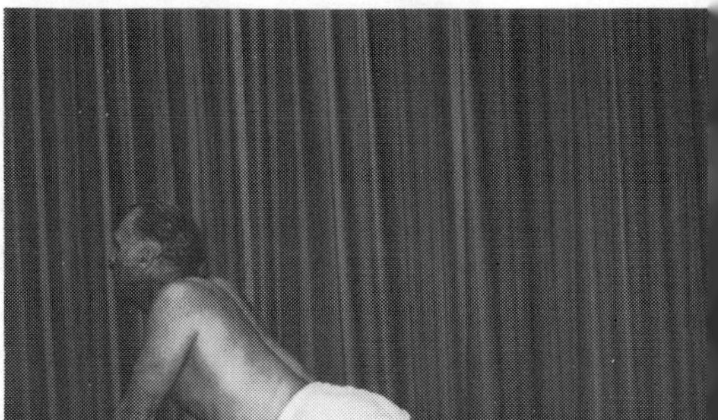

**Figure 9-5b Final position**

## EXERCISE 2: THE LOWER TRUNK STRETCHER (FRONT)

Figure 9-6c shows the final position to work toward. Figures 9-6a and 9-6b show two intermediate steps. This position will be difficult to attain for most men and for some women. However, constant practice will result in attainment of at least the second intermediate step, although it may require a period of several months of diligent effort. The results in better spinal mobility and freedom from pain are well worthwhile. Because this position is difficult, everyone should go through the intermediate steps as described.

**Intermediate Step 1**

You will require a belt or small bath towel and two sofa cushions totaling about 6 inches in thickness.

**1)** Kneel on the middle of the two cushions.

**2)** Place the belt around the lower legs.

**3)** Lie on your abdomen with the knees raised by the cushions and reach back to grasp the belt with both hands (first one hand and then both).

**4)** Pull with the belt as you press back with the lower legs to bring about a small arch in the back as shown in the figure.

**5)** Hold this 10-15 seconds the first day and gradually work up to one minute.

**6)** Breathe naturally in this position.

**Intermediate Step 2**

You will need only the belt or towel. Repeat the procedure as in Intermediate Step 1 but use more pressure with the arms and legs to arch the back without the cushions for the knees to rest upon. Again, gradually work up to holding the position for one minute.

**The Final Position: Step 3 (Figure 9-6c)**

**1)** Lie flat on the abdomen.

**2)** Bend the knees as fully as possible.

**3)** Reach back with first one hand and then the other to grasp the ankles.

**4)** Keeping the arms straight and head up, try to extend the knee joint, thus pressing the back into an arched position as in Figure 9-6c. Strive to get the knees as high as possible.

**5)** Breathe naturally and hold 10-15 seconds the first day on this step, gradually increasing to one minute.

**6)** Release very slowly and gently.

Benefits: This position has all the benefits of Exercise 1. In addition, it strengthens and tones the lower back muscles and buttocks, while stretching the hip flexors and the muscles on the front of the thighs.

**THE LOWER TRUNK STRETCHER**
**(Front)**

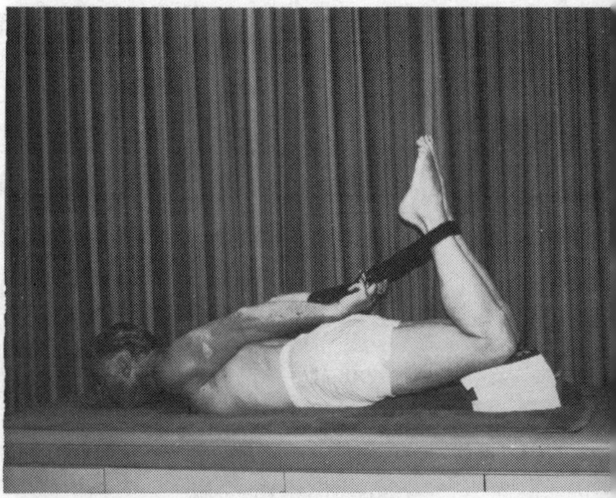

**Figure 9-6a Intermediate Step 1: with belt and cushions.**

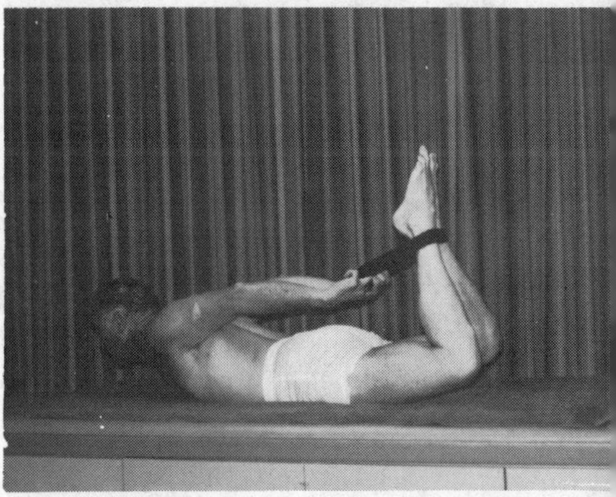

**Figure 9-6b Intermediate Step 2: with belt only.**

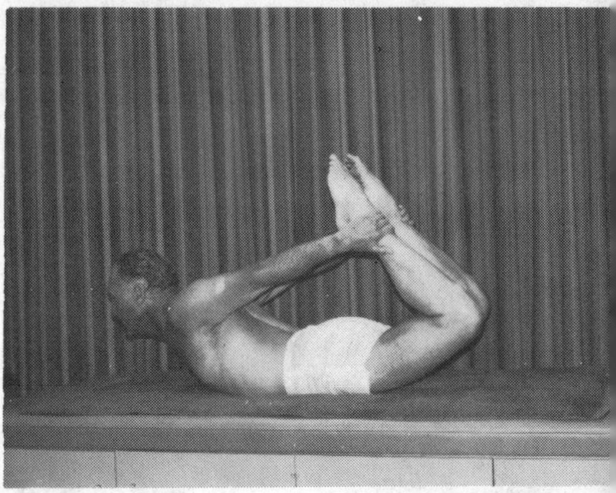

**Figure 9-6c Final position.**

## EXERCISE 3: THE UPPER BACK STRETCHER

Figure 9-7b shows the final position. This position is easy for most people to approximate and therefore only one intermediate position (and that one of degree only) is provided in Figure 9-7a. The Upper Back Stretcher is a preparatory device used by the author to bring about better results in the following exercise, number 4.

**1)** Kneel on the floor with toes pointed so that weight is borne on the entire front surface of shins and insteps, keeping buttocks in contact with calves.

**2)** Bend forward and attempt to place your head so that the scalp is on the floor, with your forehead in contact with your knees.

**3)** Stretch the arms forward until the elbows are straight and the palms of the hands are on the floor.

**4)** Hold the position 10-15 seconds the first day and increase gradually to one minute. Maintain normal (slow, easy) breathing throughout.

### Intermediate Step

The only intermediate step necessary in achieving the final position is that of allowing several inches between head and knees. However, one should always strive for the final position.

**Benefits:** This position results in stretching the muscles and connective tissues of the upper back, particularly those of the cervical and thoracic regions. The extension of the arms overhead in this position results in a very fine stretch of the latissimus dorsi and associated muscles which constitute a large proportion of the total muscle tissue of the upper back. It is the ideal preparation for Exercise 4.

### THE UPPER BACK STRETCHER

Figure 9-7a Intermediate position

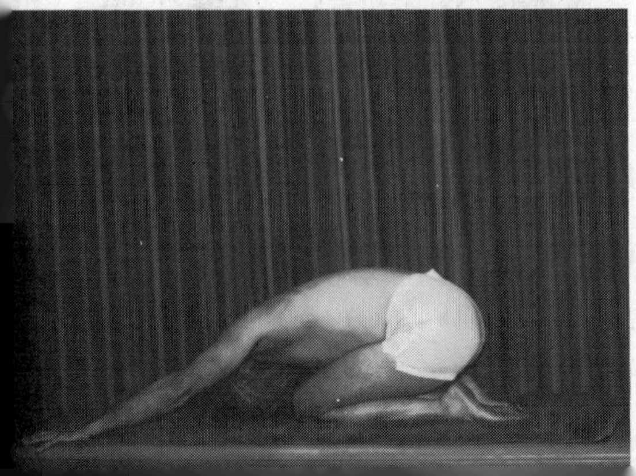

Figure 9-7b Final position

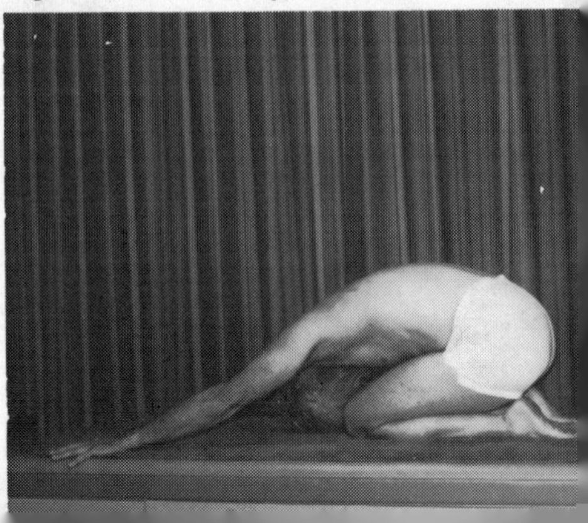

## EXERCISE 4: THE UPPER AND LOWER BACK STRETCHER

Figure 9-8d shows the final position to be achieved by the very flexible ladies. Very few older people can achieve this—especially not the men. Work for this end only if it is easy for you. Figure 9-8c shows a more realistic goal for most older people, and even this will require months of patient and persistent effort for most. Figures 9-8a and 9-8b show intermediate steps which should be used in the progression toward the position in 9-8c or 9-8d.

**Intermediate Step 1** (Figure 9-8a)

You will require a belt or small bath towel.

**1)** Sit on the floor with legs extended, feet together, and knees straight (locked out).

**2)** Loop the belt (or towel) around the feet.

**3)** Pulling on the belt with your hands, stretch, trying to bring your head as close to your feet as possible without bending the knees. *At no time should the knees be bent.* Use a greater length of belt in preference to cheating by bending the knees, because bending the knees changes the entire exercise anatomically.

**4)** Enter the position very gently and *do not, under any circumstances, bounce your body in this position!*

**5)** Hold the position for a few seconds then release the position *very slowly and gently!*

**6)** Repeat three times.

**7)** Over a period of days or weeks, work up to a one-minute period held once in this position.

**Intermediate Step 2** (Figure 9-8b)

Follow the same steps and procedures as in Intermediate Step 1, except that now discard the belt and grasp your ankles.

**Final Position**

Figure 9-8c shows the final position for most persons while Figure 9-8d illustrates the final position for the unusually flexible person. The procedure is again identical to that in the first step, but now the outer borders of the feet are grasped and held. The unusually flexible also will rest the head on the knees while the elbows rest on the ground.

**Benefits:** This exercise position stretches every muscle in the back part of the body from head to toe. Because these muscles are often overly fatigued from poor posture which may be the result of either habit or occupation, they are very often the site of small muscle spasms which can bring about the excruciating pain of the "low back syndrome." Our research using electromyographic techniques has shown how this can come about.[1] The stretching of this exercise evokes nervous reflexes which relax all of these muscles and have a strong preventive effect against muscle spasm.[2]

**A Word of Caution, However:** It is possible to put the back muscles into spasm if bouncing is resorted to while these muscles are on stretch. A too vigorous entry into the position is, of course, akin to bouncing. Therefore, I repeat: *Enter and release* from this position *very slowly and gently* and do not be overzealous in the degree to which you stretch. At no time should you stretch beyond the point of mild discomfort. *Pain has no place in our program.* The results will come slowly and surely if you do not attempt to hurry them!

**THE UPPER AND LOWER BACK STRETCHER**

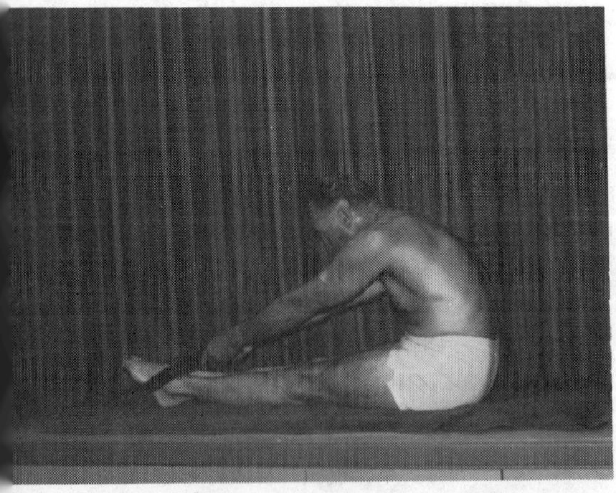

**Figure 9-8a** Intermediate Step 1: using belt.

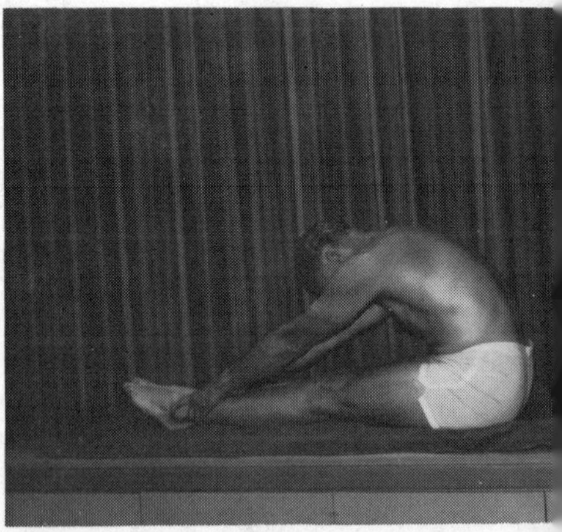

**Figure 9-8b** Intermediate Step 2: grabbin[g] ankles.

THE UPPER AND LOWER BACK STRETCHER

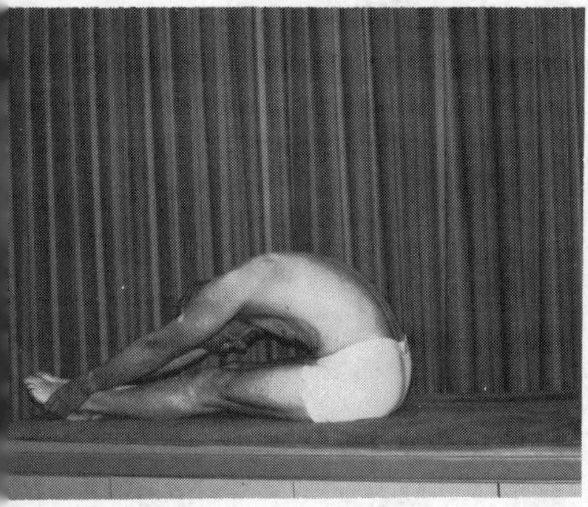

Figure 9-8c My suggested final position: grabbing feet.

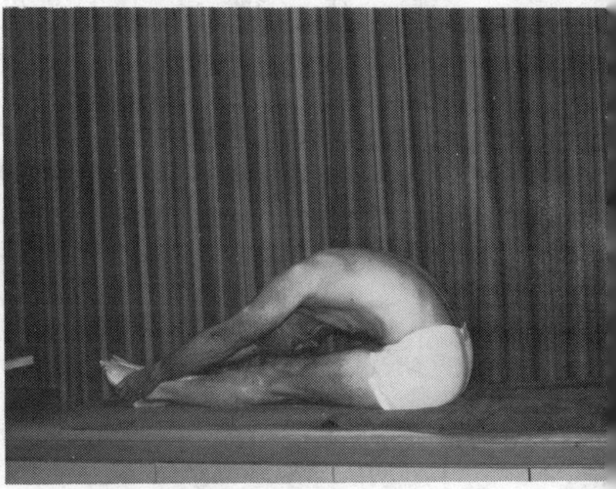

Figure 9-8d Head on knees.

## EXERCISE 5: THE NECK STRETCHER

Figure 9-9c shows the final position toward which you will direct your efforts. This is another exercise in which the final position may not be achieved easily. However, the intermediate positions are not too difficult and will start you on your way to better flexibility.

Intermediate Step 1 (Figure 9-9a)

You will need a footstool to aid you in this step.

**1)** Lie flat on your back on the floor with the footstool about one to two feet away from the top of your head.

**2)** Raise the legs over the head and place the insteps and front of the legs on the footstool, keeping the knees straight.

**3)** Place hands on hips thus helping to keep the weight of your legs on the stool.

**4)** Hold 20-30 seconds. On succeeding days work up to one minute.

**5)** Return to original resting position by bringing legs down with knees bent to prevent a heavy fall.

Intermediate Step 2 (Figure 9-9b)

Repeat the procedure of Intermediate Step 1 but eliminate the use of the footstool. Allow more of the weight to come over the top by bending the knees as in the figure. Again, work up from 20-30 seconds to one minute.

**Final Position (Figure 9-9c)**

In the final position, it is necessary only to modify Intermediate Step 2 by placing the hands at the side palm down at the start and leaving them in place as you press down with your hands to help in getting the legs overhead. More importantly, *the legs must now remain straight at the knee with the toes pointed.* Progression again goes from 20-30 seconds up to one minute in time held.

**Benefits:** This position primarily stretches the muscles of the neck and the hamstrings. Both areas are frequent sites of stiffness, aches, and pains. Maintaining good mobility in these joints lessens the incidence of such aches and pains, and may provide complete relief.

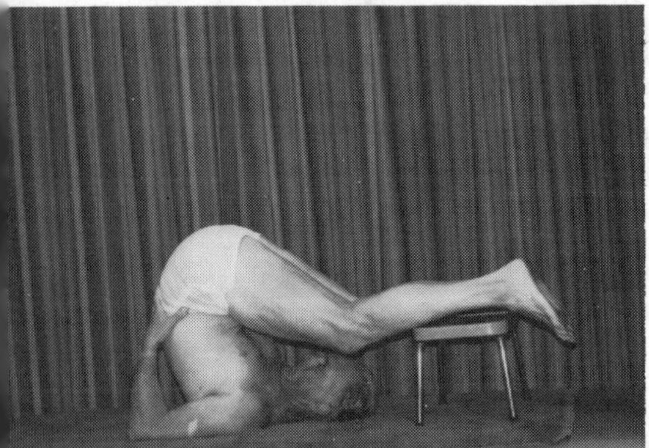

THE NECK STRETCHER

Figure 9-9a Intermediate Step 1: legs straight, feet on footstool, hands on hips.

Figure 9-9b Intermediate Step 2: no footstool, legs bent at knees, hands on hips.

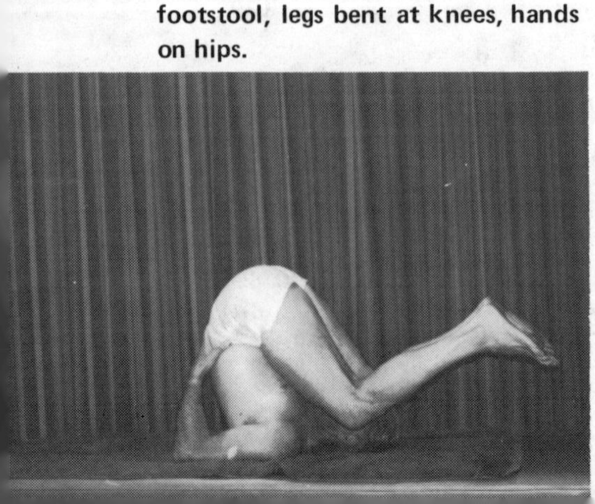

Figure 9-9c Final position

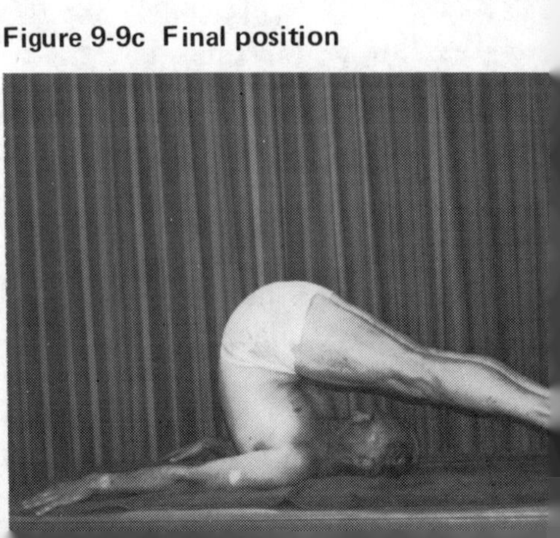

## EXERCISE 6: THE TRUNK TWISTER

Figure 9-10c shows three views of the final position we strive for. Again, the final position is difficult in the beginning, so I will provide you two relatively easy intermediate steps which will help you on your way to the final accomplishment.

**Intermediate Step 1**
(Figure 9-10a)

**1)** Start in sitting position with legs out straight and together.

**2)** Bring your right foot over your left knee and place it flat on the floor alongside the left knee.

**3)** Turn your head and shoulders to the right as far as possible, while, with your left hand, grasping your left leg below the knee.

**4)** Place your right hand on the floor behind you as far as possible to the left of your buttocks.

**5)** Hold the position (breathing normally) for 10-15 seconds the first day and work toward one minute as your progress permits.

**6)** Repeat the procedure in the other direction.

**Intermediate Step 2**
(Figure 9-10b)

**1)** Start in sitting position as for Intermediate Step 1.

**2)** Bend the left knee as fully as possible (without pain), bringing the left foot under the right leg. If possible, you should find your left heel under your right buttock, but this is not essential if your knee joint is stiff. Now, your lower leg is folded against the thigh.

**3)** Bring your right foot over your left knee and place it flat on the floor alongside the left knee.

**4)** Now reach across your right leg with the left arm to grasp your left knee with your left hand with the back of the left arm resting on the outside of the right knee.

**5)** Turn head and shoulders as far to the right as possible.

**6)** Place your right hand on the floor behind you as far as possible to the left of your buttocks.

**7)** Hold the position 10-15 seconds the first day and work toward one minute.

**8)** Repeat the procedure in the other direction.

**Final Position** (Figure 9-10c)

**1)** Start in sitting position as in Intermediate Steps 1 and 2.

**2)** Same as in Intermediate Step 2.

**3)** Same as in Intermediate Step 2.

**4)** Now grasp the ankle of your right leg with your left hand instead of grasping your left knee.

**5)** Turn head and shoulders as far to the *right* as possible.

**6)** Instead of placing your right hand on the floor, bring it around behind your back as far as possible to place your fingers palm down on your left groin.

**7)** Hold the position 10-15 seconds the first day and work toward one minute.

**8)** Repeat the procedure in the opposite direction.

**Benefits:** Because the muscles of your trunk do not all run in lengthwise directions, we must stretch those which run diagonally by twisting the trunk. Thus, in this exercise, the lower part of the trunk and spine is locked in one direction while effort is directed toward rotating the upper parts as far as possible in the opposite direction. This exercise helps to keep the muscles of the trunk and particularly those concerned with spinal rotation in a good, supple condition. This in turn helps to produce good posture, and that muscle balance which is essential to relief of backache.

**THE TRUNK TWISTER**

**Figure 9-10a Intermediate Step 1**

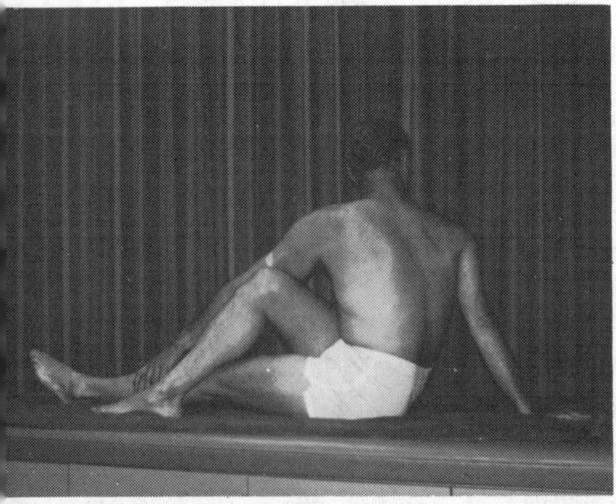

**Figure 9-10b Intermediate Step 2**

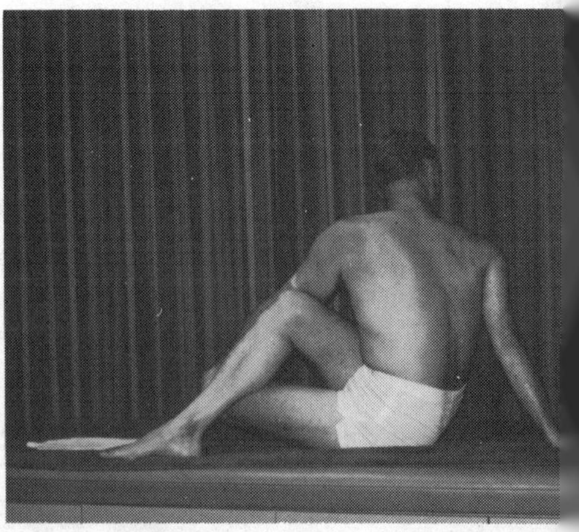

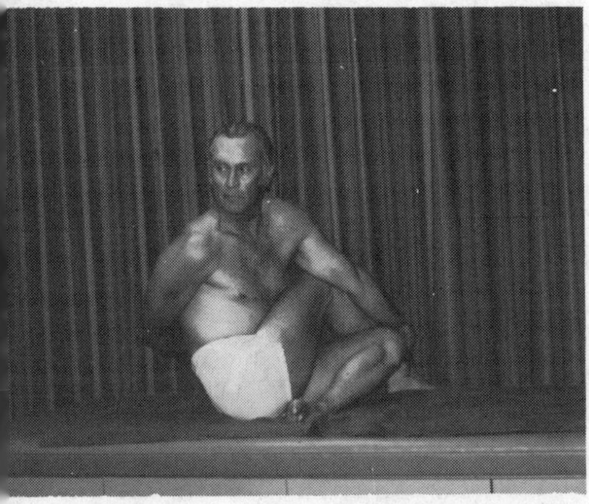

Figure 9-10c1 Right side

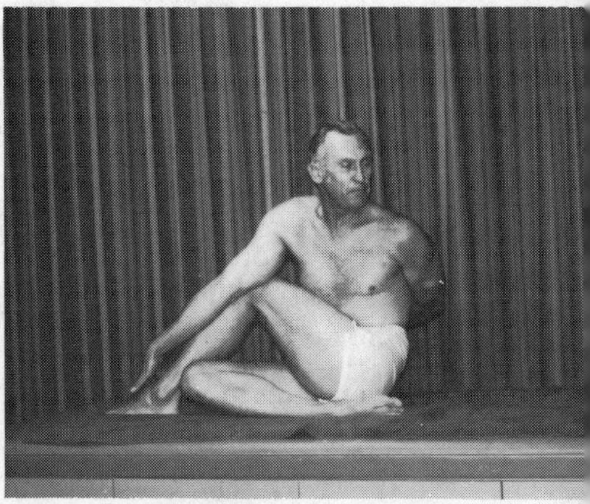

Figure 9-10c2 Left side

THE TRUNK TWISTER: FINAL POSITION

Figure 9-10c3 Back view

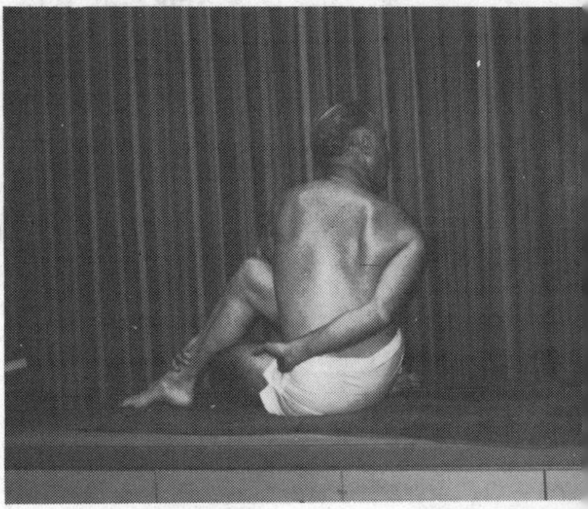

## EXERCISE 7: THE TOE POINTER

(For prevention and/or relief of shin splints)

Figure 9-11c shows the final position. Although this exercise is not extremely difficult, I will provide two intermediate positions which will form useful steppingstones for those who are quite inflexible.

**Intermediate Step 1**

(Figure 9-11a)

**1)** Kneel on the floor feet together, with the toes extended behind.

**2)** Place your hands on the floor alongside your knees and rock your weight onto the insteps sufficiently to feel the pressure in the ankles and in the muscles on the front of the lower leg.

**3)** Hold the position 10-15 seconds, and on succeeding days work toward one minute.

**4)** When one-minute duration can be accomplished, move on to Intermediate Step 2.

**Intermediate Step 2**

(Figure 9-11b)

**1)** Kneel on the floor as in Intermediate Step 1, but place the hands on the floor behind you so you can catch your weight on your hands.

**2)** Rock your weight back so that most of your weight rests over the feet.

**3)** Hold for 15-20 seconds and work up to one minute on succeeding days.

**4)** When one minute can be accomplished, move on to the final step.

**Final Position**

(Figure 9-11c)

**1)** Kneel on the floor as in Intermediate Step 2 but rock your weight gently backward until your weight comes back far enough to bring your knees off the ground.

**2)** Hold the position for 5-10 seconds. Gradually work up to one minute.

**A Word of Caution:** If you have any knee problems or any history of them, consult your physician before attempting this exercise.

**Benefits:** Many people develop pain in the front of the lower legs which can become severe after vigorous walking or jogging. This stretching exercise done after such activity will prevent the pain, often called "shin splints." The exercise also will help relieve shin splints when they already have been brought about by overly severe use of the lower legs.[3]

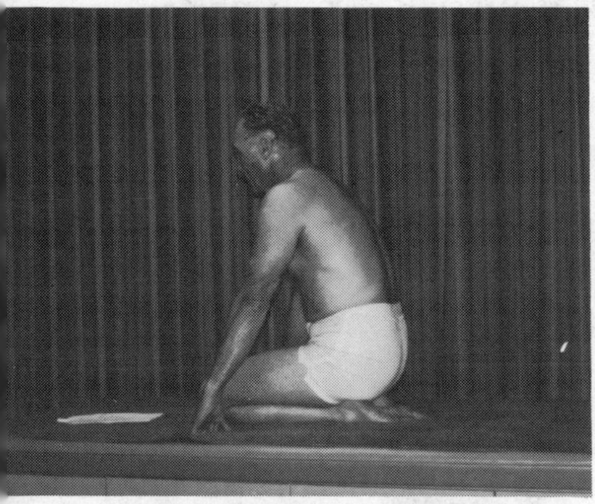

Figure 9-11a Intermediate Step 1: hands at sides, knees on ground.

THE TOE POINTER

Figure 9-11b Intermediate Step 2: hands behind, knees on ground.

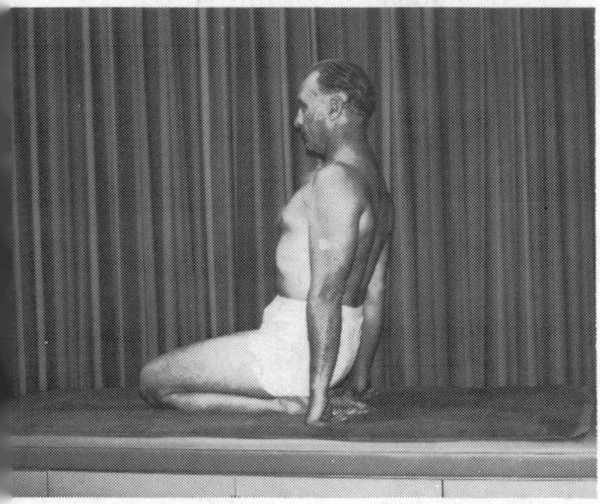

Figure 9-11c Final position: knees off floor.

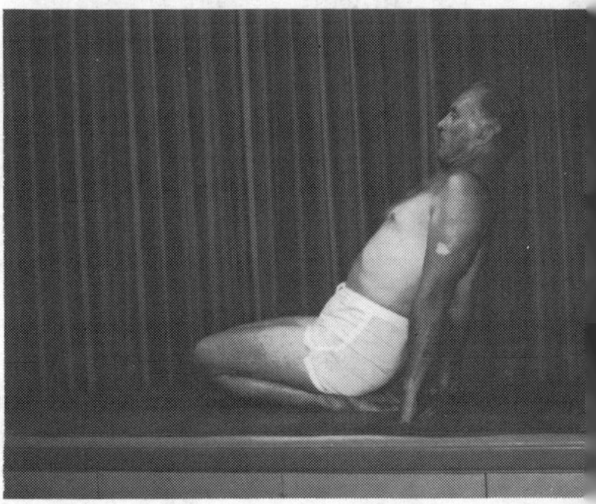

## EXERCISE 8: THE CALF AND SHOULDER STRETCHER

You will need a doorway with unobstructed wall space on each side, as shown in Figure 9-12.

**1)** Stand facing the doorway with feet shoulder-width apart and about one foot from the doorway. Keep feet pointed straight forward.

**2)** Extend the arms horizontally, straight at the elbow.

**3)** Lean forward slowly, resting your upper body weight on your arms against the walls, while allowing your head and upper body to enter the doorway. Your weight will be resting on your forearms or upper arms (depending on your width and the width of the doorway).

**4)** Keep the arms straight at the elbows, and make fists with the hands, keeping the backs of the hands pointing upward. Keep the knees and body straight throughout the exercise with heels on the floor.

**5)** Hold briefly for 5-10 seconds the first day and gradually work up to one minute.

Further progression is gained by placing the feet farther and farther from the wall. Thus, when one minute can be sustained easily with feet at 12 inches from the wall, the next step will be to attempt 18 inches for 10-15 seconds and again gradually work up to one minute, and so forth.

**Benefits:** One of the common complaints after unaccustomed brisk walking or jogging is a persistent soreness in the muscles of the calf. This exercise will prevent that soreness. It improves the suppleness of your lower leg muscles and the elasticity of the connective tissues around the ankle joint.

Further, as we grow older, we use the arms and shoulder joints less and less throughout the full range of motion. Many of us develop ill-defined aches and pains in the shoulder as a result, and shrug them off as being "bursitis." The author has found that for many such individuals the pain can be relieved by this exercise and the following one, Exercise 9.
*However, if the shoulder problem has been identified as a true bursitis by a physician then the physician should be consulted before using Exercises 8 and 9 for this purpose.*

As a matter of fact, the author designed this exercise

as an attempt to alleviate his own "bursitis." The attempt was completely successful in relieving a lifelong problem, which previous treatments had not helped!

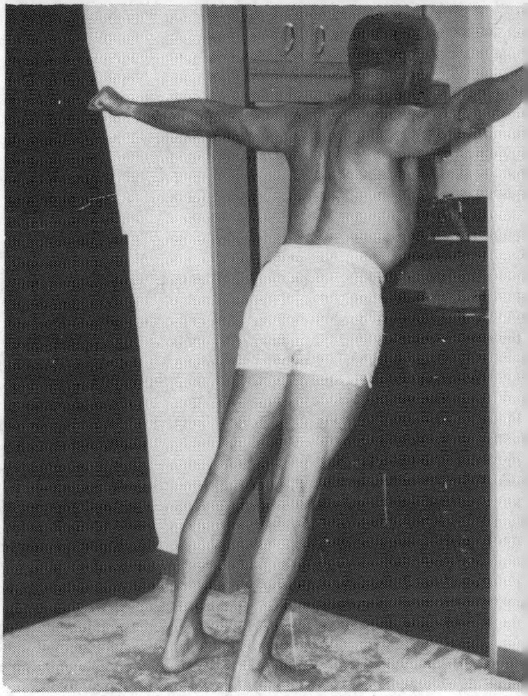

**Figure 9-12 THE CALF AND SHOULDER STRETCHER**

## EXERCISE 9: THE SHOULDER AND BICEPS STRETCHER

For this exercise (see Figure 9-13), you will need a dresser, a bookshelf, or some other piece of furniture with a top that is at, or only slightly below, your shoulder level.

**1)** Stand with your back to the dresser about one foot away from it, with your feet shoulder-width apart.

**2)** Interlace your fingers behind your back, clasping your hands palm to palm.

**3)** Bend forward at the waist, allowing your arms to come up easily behind you, and place your hands on the bookshelf or dresser top.

**4)** Straighten the body *slowly and gently* until *mild discomfort* is felt in the arms and/or shoulders.

**5)** Hold this position 5-10 seconds. On successive days work toward the one-minute goal.

Progression is provided by working toward standing more and more erect until you reach the position shown in Figure 9-13. If you are quite flexible, you may even eventually need to raise the height of the hands by placing a book or two on the shelf or dresser top.

**Benefits:** This exercise provides a static stretch for the biceps muscle, which otherwise is very difficult to stretch. It also stretches the part of the deltoid (shoulder) muscle which often becomes painful as the result of unusual movements. This exercise together with Exercise 8 will provide relief from the minor but annoying shoulder pains experienced by so many older people.

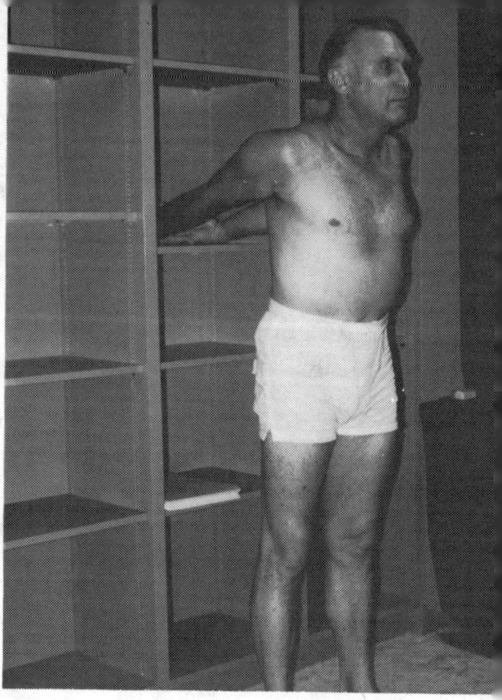

Figure 9-13 THE SHOULDER AND BICEPS STRETCHER

**This Concludes Your Level I Exercise Program Now—You Can Shower!**

**Retesting and Advancement to Level II**

At the end of the first six weeks at Level I you will retest yourself on the Progressive Pulse Rate Test to observe your progress. If you are now at the "above average" level on all four stepping rates, you are ready for advancement to Level II even though you might not have completed all the steps of the progressive walking program. If you score in at least the "average" category on all four stepping rates *and* have completed the entire progressive walking program without exceeding the limit heart rate of 120, then you may also proceed to Level II.

If you do not yet satisfy either of these criteria (*or* if your physician wishes you to remain on Level I), you will continue the program of Level I until a later six-weeks' retest meets the criteria. Do not be impatient, because even the Level I program brings about very significant improvement in fitness for older people.

# 10

# EXERCISE PRESCRIPTION

## Level II

Congratulations!

By the time you are ready to enter this stage of your exercise program, you are well along the road to levels of physical fitness that will enhance the pleasure of living.

Level II consists of the same three phases as Level I, except that in Level II, you will begin the jog-walk program as a substitute for the progressive walking of Level I. The second phase of Level II consists of the same calisthenics, except that now you will be doing more repetitions in each two-minute period. The third phase, static stretching, remains the same. No advancement beyond the final positions noted in Level I are necessary, so there will be no changes described in this chapter. It is to be hoped (although not expected for all) that by now you can accomplish the full one-minute period of each stretching exercise at the final position. If this is not the case, you will simply continue as described in Chapter 9. By no means should you discontinue the static stretching exercises. You should continue doing them at the advanced levels (after you can comfortably achieve them) henceforward as the final cooling down phase of your lifelong physical fitness program.

Before embarking on the jog-walk phase of Level II, you will want to refer back to Chapter 8 to refresh your memory on details such as equipment needed and measurement of the course.

## FIRST PHASE—THE JOG-WALK PROGRAM

In this phase, your ultimate goal is the improvement of your heart, lungs, and muscles to the point that you can jog one mile without stopping, and do it *easily—without strain.* You will work progressively toward this goal by alternating a given number of steps jogged with a given number of steps walked. Please note that I do not set the jogging *rate* for you. Rate or speed is the chief determinant of the activity's stressfulness. Therefore, you are to set your own rate at a level which is *comfortable* for you.

What is jogging, and how does it differ from running? "Jogging" is a rather poorly defined term. It means different things to different people. For our purposes, we will take the term to mean a "slow trot," which constitutes the first step up from walking toward running. The term "running" implies speed; and we are not at all interested in speed. Because jogging is just one level above walking, technique or "form" is not so important as it is for the young track athlete trying to set a new record. However, a few words might be in order to improve your efficiency and to prevent unnecessary problems from arising.

First, posture should be considered. Jog with the head up and body erect; otherwise, you cannot fully expand the lungs. Secondly, in the interests of efficiency, you must "stay loose." Don't tense up or force yourself in any way. Jogging must be done easily, naturally and *without strain.* Thirdly, keep all movements in the forward-backward direction, and eliminate any tendency toward crosswise movements. These literally are at cross-purposes to your goal. Your feet should be pointed straight ahead. You can check this easily by observing your footprints on sand or soft ground, or on pavement after jogging through a puddle. Also, your arms should be allowed to swing easily in rhythm with your leg motion, forward-backward, not across your body.

The way the feet strike the ground varies from person to person. In fast running, it is necessary to run on the ball of the foot. But in the slower jogging, most people find it most natural to bring the whole foot into contact with the gound. Most find it natural to bring the foot down, heel first, then toe. But some prefer to contact the ball of the foot first, then the full foot. In any event, do what comes naturally for you. Don't let undue concern for technique interfere with the relaxation and pleasure of jogging.

Fourth, a word about breathing. Up to this point in the program, normal breathing through the nose has been both possible and desirable. However, the demands for air (actually oxygen) in jogging exceed what can be delivered through nose-breathing alone. Therefore, you will find it necessary to breathe through the mouth and the nose in order to meet the new demand for oxygen. It is this very challenge to your respiratory system, of course, which brings about the eventual response of deeper and better breathing capacity which I discussed earlier. This is one of the most important health benefits of our program.

One final observation regarding the footwear for jogging: Buy only good quality tennis shoes with a thick, resilient sole, or jogging shoes. In either case they should fit a bit more snugly than your street shoes so that your foot cannot slip or slide within the shoe. If the eyelets for the laces come closer to each other than about one inch, the shoes probably are cut too wide for your foot. You should select another brand which is cut better for you. However, it is obvious that the shoes also must not be too tight for comfort. Fit is very important in preventing blisters and other foot discomfort. Probably you will be more likely to get qualified assistance in this matter from sales people in sporting goods stores rather than those in general department stores or shoe stores.

Weather also must be considered. In those parts of the country where protracted periods of seriously inclement weather can be expected, substitutions are necessary for first phase activities, at least at Level II. The progressive walking program usually can be carried on in most parts of the country by the simple expedient of changing the schedule to concentrate the exercises into those days in which walking remains possible. For example, a whole week stretch or more of really impossible weather could be followed by walking every day until the schedule is regained.

However, this remedy is not always possible for the jog-walk program. Ice and/or snow might make jogging not only difficult but possibly dangerous. In this case, there are several substitutions. First, the jogging can be done "in place" and the walk phase can be done up and down a hallway. Jogging in place is not quite so strenuous as the real thing but this will not seriously throw you off your schedule.

A second alternative is the use of your testing stool to do stool-stepping at a rate and for a duration roughly equivalent to your point in the jog-walk progression. To do this, you will go back to the results of your most recent PPR Test and select that rate of bench-stepping which evoked a heart rate response most similar to that which you have recorded for your last day's jog-walk workout. Do this by dividing the two-minute recovery pulse rate of the PPR by two and adding 20 beats per minute to the result. This will give a rough approximation of the heart rate achieved during the stepping and will allow you to select the proper stepping rate. Because 50 steps of jogging take approximately 20 seconds, you will do the bench-stepping for 20 seconds. Take your heart rate and walk the appropriate number of steps (depending on your current point of progress in the program) for your walk interval so that the end of the walk will place you back at the stepping stool again for the next set of jog-walk.

Another possible substitution is to use rope-skipping, but this is recommended only for those who have some skill at this activity. Further, it must be done by trial and error until the heart rate response to various paces and methods of rope-skipping has been established.

In general, the "game plan" for your jog-walk program revolves around another "double progressive" training procedure. That is, you will start with only a very modest challenge to your cardiovascular and respiratory systems, initially modifying only distance jogged, and later modifying the intensity by shortening the rest periods (walking). This system has been shown to work very well both in laboratory experiments and in practical experience with older people.

Each day, you will perform from five to ten sets of jog-walk. Each set consists of a given number of steps jogged, and a given number of steps walked to provide the rest interval. The first day you will do 5 sets of 50 steps jog and 50 steps walk. The second day, you will do 6 sets, the third day 7 sets, and so on, until you have completed 10 sets of 50 jog, 50 walk.

Up to this point, your progression has been achieved by increasing duration or distance. As I pointed out earlier, distance progression is very gentle, in that it makes only a very small increase in demands on your heart and lungs.

Having completed 10 sets of 50-50, now you are ready to progress by increasing the intensity of your exercise. This can be done by either moving faster or by cutting down the rest, which is the walk interval. The latter is the safer course, so you now jog 50 steps but walk only 40. However, you also go back to doing only 5 sets. The entire progression is shown in Table 10-1:

**TABLE 10-1: JOG-WALK PROGRAM**

1) 50 steps jog, 50 steps walk
    a) 5 sets the first day
    b) Each day increase the number of sets by one until 10 sets have been completed
    c) Use the same set procedure for each new series of jog-walk
2) 50 steps jog, 40 steps walk
3) 50 steps jog, 30 steps walk
4) 50 steps jog, 20 steps walk
5) 50 steps jog, 10 steps walk
6) 75 steps jog, 10 steps walk
7) 100 steps jog, 10 steps walk
8) 125 steps jog, 10 steps walk
9) 150 steps jog, 10 stesp walk
10) 175 steps jog, 10 steps walk
11) 200 steps jog, 10 steps walk
12) Individual program

Throughout the jog-walk program if you are in your fifties or sixties, you are to set yourself a "limit heart rate" of 140 beats per minute. If you are 70 or older, the limit heart rate is 130 beats per minute. By so doing, you will stay below about 85 percent of your maximum. This level is very effective in terms of training for the healthy older person, without danger of overstress.

You will take your heart rate immediately at the end of each 50-step jog interval. So long as it remains below "limit rate" you will stay with the progression outlined in Table 10-1.

If you exceed the limit rate, you might be jogging too fast. If this is not the case, you will increase the walk interval by 10 steps and then return to the appropriate point of progression in Table 10-1.

You will arrive at "individual program," the final step of Table 10-1, in about six months' time if you train three times per week at an average rate of progress. You then will take the next step, which is to jog steadily for one-quarter mile, at the end of which you will check your heart rate. So long as you remain under "limit rate" you may now increase your jogging distance by one-eighth mile as the spirit moves you, until you reach the ultimate goal of one mile continuous jogging without rest, and without exceeding the limit heart rate.

After completing all the sets of jog-walk or continuous jogging on any given workout day, it is important to walk for an additional two to three minutes or more. This will provide your system a gradual "cooling down" from the vigorous exercise to the resting state. More about the importance of this in Chapter 12.

When you first achieve one mile of continuous jogging, you will find that your time for this distance will vary between 9 and 12 minutes, depending on your age and lifetime history of physical activity. Some older men who have pursued marathon running throughout their lifetimes can, of course, do far better than nine minutes for a mile, but this is not necessary to achieve optimal levels of health and physical fitness. If you happen to be the very competitive type who shoots for maximum performance, I suggest that you *revisit your physician* before attempting to do any better than a nine-minute mile.

Now that we have reviewed the general game plan, you are ready for the first day in Level II. You will need your stopwatch (or watch with sweep second hand) and a small clipboard with pencil, plus your copy of Table E, presented in the Appendix. If you must walk some distance to and from a suitable jogging course, so much the better.

Because jogging itself is an excellent warm-up, you will start out with 50 steps jogging. At the end of 50 steps jogging, you will take your heart rate. At first, you will need to stop to take your heart rate. But most of you will arrive at the point that you can get it during the walk interval. You will walk 50 steps and then immediately begin the second set of 50 jog-50 walk. On the first day you will complete five sets, taking your heart rate and recording it after each jog. It is important that you take the heart rate as quickly as possible after ending the jog interval.

If you exceeded the limit heart rate (130 or 140, depending on your age) on the first day, you will need to add 10 steps to the walk interval. Thus, on the second day, you do five sets of 50 jog-60 walk, and progress from there. At any step in the progression where you consistently hit the limit heart rate, you should then spend an extra day (or even several days) at the same step without further advance on the progression. Remember, you need not be slavish about adherence to the progression—the important factor is that your circulatory system makes the desirable responses *without undue stress. Time is not a factor.*

Table 10-2 gives the estimated heart rate responses to various levels of jog-walk, according to physical fitness level. It is designed specifically to determine the appropriate starting level of jog-walk for those who found the 50 jog-50 walk set too easy on the first day, as indicated by heart rate considerably below 130; and for those who scored "excellent" or "very good" on the PPR Test.

**TABLE 10-2: MAXIMUM HEART RATE IN FIVE SETS***

| Fitness Category (PPR Test) | 50 jog 50 walk | 50 jog 40 walk | 50 jog 30 walk | 50 jog 20 walk | 50 jog 10 walk |
|---|---|---|---|---|---|
| Excellent | 110 (102-118) | 115 (107-123) | 119 (111-127) | 122 (114-130) | 126 (118-134) |
| Very Good | 113 (105-121) | 118 (110-126) | 122 (114-130) | 124 (116-132) | 128 (120-136) |
| Average | 117 (109-125) | 122 (114-130) | 125 (117-133) | 128 (120-136) | 133 (125-141) |
| Below Average | 122 (114-130) | 126 (118-134) | 130 (122-138) | 132 (124-140) | 137 (129-145) |
| Poor | 126 (118-134) | 128 (120-136) | 132 (124-140) | 135 (127-143) | 140 (132-148) |

*These data were established in the author's laboratory by radiotelemetry methods. The upper figure represents the average heart rate response. The lower figures represent the range for plus or minus one standard deviation.

Here's an example of how the table is used to determine your starting level if the 50 steps jog, 50 steps walk was too easy: If you're in your fifties or sixties, and you scored "average" on the PPR Test, you can safely enter the program at 50 steps jog, 20 steps walk. This is so because your most likely heart rate response will be about 128 beats per minute; and the odds are two to one that that rate will be between 120 and 136. Notice that I have been very conservative in advising all who were average or below to start on Level I. This was to provide a large safety factor in the event of inaccuracies in heart rate count. It also should have prevented you from developing sore muscles, blisters, or other problems if you have been quite sedentary through life.

Another example: If you scored "excellent" or "very good" on the PPR Test, you'll note that the table indicates that five sets of 50 jog steps, 10 walk steps should give you a comfortable workout, with the heart rate response expected to be 126 for "excellent" and 128 for "very good."

Remember, even if you determine that you should start the jog-walk program at a higher level than 50 jog-50 walk, the same general instructions and plan of progression apply to you. The only difference is your starting point. The first day, you do five sets at the appropriate level, and progress from there as outlined in Table 10-1.

## SECOND PHASE: CALISTHENICS

Your muscular strength, muscular endurance, and flexibility do not necessarily improve at the same rate as your circulatory-respiratory responses to walking and jog-walk. Even though you are ready for Level II in jogging, you must wait to advance in the second phase until you are able to achieve easily, without exceeding the Level I limit heart rate of 120, the following repetitions of calisthenics:

| | | |
|---|---|---|
| Exercise 1) | The Bender | 20 in two minutes |
| Exercise 2) | Easy Push-up | 40 in two minutes |
| Exercise 3) | Slow-Motion Flutter Kick | 20 in two minutes |
| Exercise 4) | Easy Sit-up | 40 in two minutes |

When these goals are attained, you are ready to begin the following Level II calisthenic program.

| Level II Calisthenics | Rate | Time | Total Repetition |
|---|---|---|---|
| 1) The Bender | 10-20 per min. | 2 min. | 20-40 |
| 2) Full Body Push-up | as you please | — | as many as possible without strain |
| 3) Flutter Kick | 10-20 per min. | 2 min. | 20-40 |
| 4) Full Body Sit-up | 10-20 per min. | 2 min. | 20-40 |

## EXERCISE 1: THE BENDER

This is continued just as in Level I (Figure 9-1), but the rate is gradually increased (at will) toward a maximum of 40 in two minutes.

## EXERCISE 2: THE FULL BODY PUSH-UP (for men only)

This is a two-count exercise, as shown in Figure 10-1, a) and b). The counting is done as for The Easy Push-up (Figure 9-2) and the starting position is also the same. The only difference is that now the body remains straight from feet to shoulders, thus creating more resistance. It is important to resist doing this exercise to the point of straining. Do not hold your breath: Breathe normally. At the first sign of difficulty drop to the down position and rest.

THE FULL BODY PUSH-UP

Figure 10-1a Down position

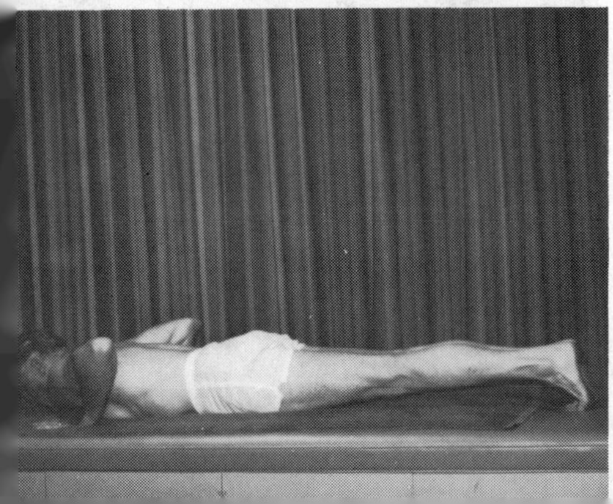

Figure 10-1b Up position

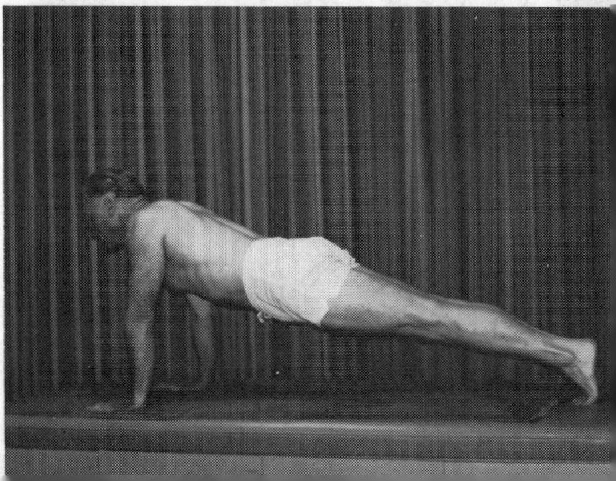

## EXERCISE 3: THE FLUTTER KICK

This is identical to Exercise 3 of Level I (Figure 9-3) except that now the cadence can be increased to a maximum of 40 in the two-minute period.

## EXERCISE 4: THE FULL BODY SIT-UP

This is a two-count exercise, as shown in Figure 10-2, a) and b). Starting position is flat on the back with hands behind neck, knees bent as shown in the figure. You may lock the feet under a piece of furniture or have a partner hold them for you, if necessary.

**Count 1:** Lift head, shoulders, and upper body off the floor and bring the right elbow to touch the left knee (alternating left elbow to right knee).

**Count 2:** Return to starting position.

**Note:** The cadence may be gradually increased up to 20 per minute for a total of 40 sit-ups for the well-conditioned older individual. More than this is neither necessary nor desirable.

**THE FULL BODY SIT-UP**

Figure 10-2a Down position

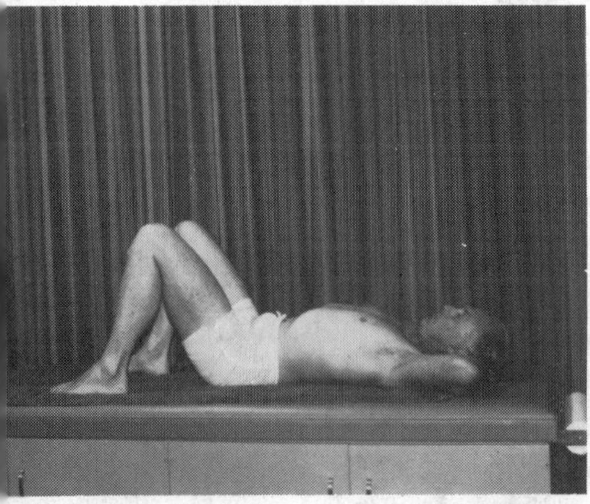

Figure 10-2b Up position

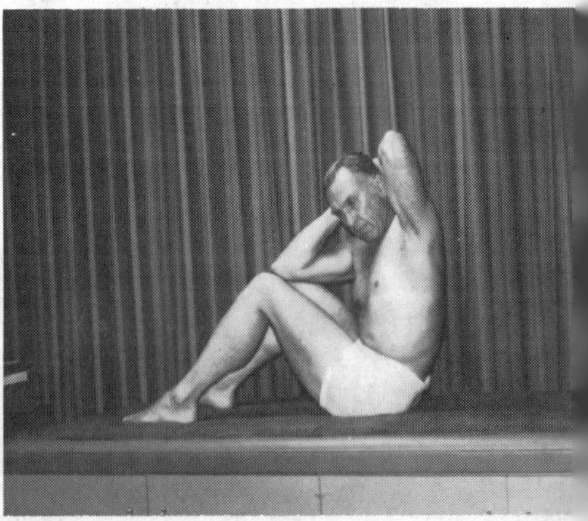

### THIRD PHASE: STATIC STRETCHING

This remains exactly as in Level I (Figures 9-5 through 9-14). The ultimate goal is still to achieve the final positions and to hold them for one minute in each case.

It will be noted that while the entire exercise program was necessarily lengthy in Level I because of the time required for the progressive walking program, it is quite streamlined in Level II and usually can be completed in 30 to 45 minutes in its entirety.

**This Concludes Your Level II Exercise Program**
**Now—You Can Shower!**

When you have arrived at the maximum levels of achievement of Level II, you have arrived at a regimen which can constitute the basic element of your lifelong physical fitness program. By continuing Level II on a regular basis with the continuing approval of your physician, you will maintain the level of fitness you have achieved, and thus maintain your new-found vigor!

# 11

# THERE'S EXERCISE . . . AND THERE'S EXCERCISE

## *Perspective*

"What you need is a little exercise. . . ."

How many times have you heard this from a well-meaning friend? Let me point out that this sort of advice is just about as meaningless as a doctor's prescription that would read "administer some drugs." The fallacy in the latter is readily apparent, because "drugs" can mean anything from strychnine to aspirin. Administering one when another is needed obviously would have dire consequences.

The same can be said about the use of exercise for health. It's true that the use of exercise for prophylactic and therapeutic purposes has not yet attained the status of drug prescriptions. Nevertheless, there is a growing body of scientific knowledge which can be used as a basis for prescription of specific exercise. When the physician prescribes a drug, he is concerned with the drug's type, the concentration of active ingredients in the preparation, and the frequency and duration of administration. In prescribing exercise, the exercise physiologist is learning to be equally concerned with the type of exercise, its intensity, and the frequency and duration of each workout.

Several years ago, when my Administration on Aging-sponsored research at the University of Southern California generated considerable publicity in the news media, one of the statements made frequently was that I was developing a "pharmacopoeia of exercise." The term capitalizes on the analogy between prescription of drugs and prescription of exercise, as we described above. However, it must be realized that the *U.S. Pharmacopoeia* is a voluminous, authoritative treatise on the preparation of drugs and their usage. It is the result of contributions by thousands of highly trained scientists. The point is, no one scientist could produce a pharmacopoeia of exercise any more than one person could have produced the *U.S. Pharmacopoeia*. However, it is my earnest hope that I, along with many other health professionals throughout the world, can contribute to a "pharmacopoeia of exercise." This is an important professional goal because such a body of knowledge is urgently needed as a health enhancement resource for people of all ages.

When I began my work with the older residents of Laguna Hills Leisure World in the USC-AOA study, the type of exercise to be used was decided on the basis of feasibility. Only calisthenics, walking, and jogging activities could conceivably be extended to widespread usage by large groups of senior citizens; and this, of course, was one of the purposes of our study. But little was known about desirable "intensity" of these exercises. At that time, scientific data were scanty even relative to young people, and virtually nothing was known of exercise "dose-response" for persons in their sixties, seventies, and eighties. For this reason, our first efforts were directed toward learning: How much exercise is enough to bring about the desired training effect? And how much is too much?

### In Pursuit of Answers

In pursuit of answers to these questions, we first brought our older subjects into the laboratory after medical screening and physiological testing and placed electrocardiographic electrodes on their chests. The electrodes' leads were connected to an FM radio transmitter about the size of a pack of cigarettes, which was strapped to the waist. The transmitter sent heart rate response data to a receiver as the subjects carried on the proposed exercises of the program. By this use of radiotelemetry, we were able to observe the subjects' responses to each activity without hampering their movements. This gave us the "dose-response" data we needed to work safely with older persons. In essence, it also provided an answer to the second question—"How much is too much?"—at least for our age group under our set of conditions.[1]

The "How much is enough?" question was answered as we trained our subjects after the actual program got under way. By relating the improvements in physical fitness to the heart rates recorded in the jog-walk program, for example, we were able to determine the lowest level that would be effective in bringing about the desired improvements.[2]

But persistent questions remained, particularly about the effects of different types of exercise. It had long been known that increasing workloads of exercise bring about increases in blood pressure. This suggested the need to evaluate these blood pressure effects in a controlled experiment with our older subjects. The level of blood pressure is an important health factor for persons of any age. Remember, the work of the heart muscle is determined almost entirely by the *pressure* against which it must pump, not by the *amount* of blood pumped. And this is particularly significant for older people.

At about the time we were completing our USC-AOA-sponsored study, some very interesting research results were published from several of the outstanding exercise physiology laboratories in Europe. There now seemed to be agreement that the *type* of exercise, at least in the young, has a great deal to do with elevation of blood pressure levels. That is, the research indicated that some types of exercise tend to create more marked and undesirable blood pressure elevation than others.

This is so, the research indicated, because different exercises require different usage of the muscles. When a muscle is in contraction, for example, the blood vessels within the tissue are "squeezed down," and high pressures are required to get the blood flow through. This localized high pressure then re-sets, to a higher level, the central mechanisms that control the general body blood pressure. The studies indicated that the most extreme blood pressure effects are generated by exercise in which small muscles are used at high proportions of their capacity,[3] and in exercise which involves isometric contractions.[4] Isometric contractions are those in which a strong contraction is maintained in a stationary position over a period of time.

Additionally, the data also indicated that in rhythmic, free-moving exercise, such as walking or jogging, each muscle contraction is followed by a period of relaxation. Consequently, there is not time for the blood pressure to build very high during contraction.

The results of our experiments with older people agreed completely with these previously published data on the young. It is clear that exercise programs for older people should be built around natural, rhythmic, free-moving patterns, such as walking, jogging, running, and swimming. Any exercise involving strong isometric contraction is to be avoided.[5]

Improvement of joint mobility is another case in which "there's exercise, and then there's exercise." Everyone who has been involved in the bouncing, jerking type of calisthenics can testify to the sore muscles that result. These sore muscles in all probability are minor local muscle spasms.[6] In older people, minor muscle spasms have a way of growing into major aches and pains. Who needs them? I have shown in a controlled experiment that the same benefits can be brought about by the *static stretching* methods which I have outlined for you in Chapter 9.[7] Most important, there is a tremendous difference physiologically between the static and the bouncing type of stretch. The *bouncing* type of stretch elicits a stretch reflex which *makes the muscle shorten* just when you are trying to force it into lengthening. You literally are working at cross-purposes. The *static stretching*, on the other hand, brings about only reflexes which relax the muscles you are trying to lengthen. Let's learn from the cat. You won't see him bouncing to accomplish the suppleness which makes his movements a thing of beauty!

### The Moral of the Story

The moral of this story, then, is that exercise should be considered in many ways to be a potent drug. Exercise, like drugs, is not to be taken indiscriminately. The type, duration, and intensity of exercise can mean the difference between potential danger and enhancement of your health and vigor!

# SEPARATING SENSE FROM NONSENSE

## A Final Word

By now, you're well aware that I have not expounded on some miraculous new method of exercise that can be considered a panacea for all ills.

Instead, I have offered a structured approach based on scientifically validated procedures. This approach has been shown to be both safe and effective for attainment of better health through physical fitness for mature men and women.

As one trained in both physical education and physiology, I would be guilty of unscientific dogmatism and parochialism if I were to imply that the methods I have described are the only ones useful for improving fitness. To be sure, there are many types of exercise which improve the function of the circulatory and respiratory systems. These include such activities as swimming, tennis, bicycling, handball, squash, and many others too numerous to mention. However, few of these lend themselves to the controlled, quantitative approach. This requires adjustments of intensity, duration, frequency, and duration of rest periods. In our program, however, we have defined the dose-response relationships to suit the needs of the unconditioned older man or woman.

Those few other physical activities which also can meet the requirements of the controlled quantitative approach have other inherent liabilities. Take swimming, for example. This is one of the finest of exercises when it is done well by a skilled swimmer. However, only a very small percentage of older men and women have the high level of skill required to swim long and far enough to bring about any real effects on heart, lungs, and circulation. Further, there are the problems of finding a suitable, uncrowded year-round facility. Finally, swimming might be contra-indicated by residual medical problems such as sinusitis or tendency to ear infections. Bicycling is another very fine conditioner, but it might be hazardous in cities, and it is impossible through long winter seasons in colder regions of the country.

For these reasons, I designed my conditioning methods around the walking and jog-walk concept so the needs of the greatest number could be served safely, effectively, and with a minimum cost for special equipment. To my knowledge, this is the only system which has been specifically developed for, and laboratory tested on, significant numbers of men and women over fifty.

To be realistic, I recognize that not all of us are possessed of the desire and/or the self-discipline necessary to pursue this sort of conditioning program as a lifelong process. I strongly recommend that the orderly regimen of our program be followed at least until you have achieved the upper levels of fitness for your age as estimated from your score on the PPR testing *and* the achievement of a one-half mile continuous jog. At this point, if you are happy with the program, make an effort to continue it. No other will provide any better results. On the other hand, if at this point you would like to revive some previously enjoyable sports skill as a *part* of your fitness program, so much the better. By now you have learned all the important methods for monitoring your safety and progress: the first by checking your heart rate and staying within the limits described in previous chapters; and the second by frequent re-checks on the PPR Test.

If you do wish to add a sports activity, here are my recommendations:

**1) Clear the proposed sports program with your physician.**

**2) Retain the program as outlined in Chapter 10 on a two-day per week basis.**

3) Do not add more than two days per week of sports activity if it is very vigorous, and not more than three days of sports activity of any sort.

4) Check your heart rate at frequent intervals in the early stages of the added program.

5) Use the static stretching exercises following the sports activity to prevent muscle soreness and to maintain mobility.

6) Check your fitness level with the PPR Test monthly for the first six months of the new activity. Any drop in the PPR score is a probable indication that you are overdoing. If this should occur, reduce the new activity to one day per week and continue the standard Level II program two days a week.

### Summary: The Sensible Procedures for Using Exercise for Health Enhancement

In bringing this book to a close, it is appropriate to reiterate the sensible procedures governing the use of exercise for health enhancement. I have alluded to most of these principles in one form or another previously, and all have been built into the Level I and Level II exercise programs. However, let me summarize the important do's and don'ts, expanding on some of the precautions, to refresh your memory so you can apply them to your lifelong fitness program, particularly in the resumption of sports activity.

**Medical Consultation and Examination:** Always re-check with your physician before making any significant changes in your physical activity pattern, particularly if such changes could make large or sudden demands on your circulatory system.

**Gradual Progress:** Always start with a low level of exertion and make progress slowly. You will notice how carefully I have led you from one step to the next in the Level I and Level II programs. You will want to take the same precautions in attempting any new activity. For example, if you wish to start playing tennis after a 20- or 30-year layoff, you do not begin by challenging the club champion. In fact, you should not start out by playing a game. Instead, you should go to a tennis club, schoolyard, or public court where a backboard is available. Here you can review your skills and practice them at a rate suitable *to you.* Take your heart rate response periodically, and *rest* at any time you reach the limit value. When comfortable fatigue sets in, *stop.* The next step would be to play "pony sets," or best three of five games, with an opponent of similar age and tennis skills. Later, playing one set of doubles with opponents of similar caliber would be appropriate.

**Your Own Limit:** Know your limit and stay well within it. Generally, you are overdoing if any one of the following applies: your exercise heart rate is above limit value as defined earlier; your sleep is not as sound as usual; or you are fatigued on the day following your workout.

**Frequency of Workouts:** Although the evidence is not yet conclusive, it is probable that best results will be gained by a minimum of three and a maximum of five workouts per week. After achieving peak condition, muscular benefits can be maintained by as little as one workout per week. But it is doubtful that once a week will maintain your cardiovascular fitness.

**Duration of Workouts:** It appears that a minimum of about 20 minutes is sufficient if the exercise intensity is high—well above 40 percent of heart rate range. However, for older people, a longer workout (up to 60 minutes or more) with a lighter intensity is a safer procedure in the earlier stages. That is the reason, of course, that our Level I program is built around walking.

**Warming up:** It is essential to the welfare of older persons' muscles, bones, joints, and ligaments that any workout begin with exercise designed to bring about *gradual* increases in blood flow with concomitant increases in local tissue and general body temperature. This is a necessity for prevention of muscular aches, pains, and injuries. Generally, no very vigorous movements should be made until sweating has begun. For example, before playing tennis, in which you frequently must lunge or reach for "hard to get" balls, warm-up should be accomplished by jogging until sweating occurs. Muscles and connective tissues are most easily injured when they are cold. The older we get, the more important the warm-up procedure becomes.

**Cooling Down:** The need to make a gradual transition from vigorous exercise back to the resting state is as important as warming up because of the adjustments the circulatory system must make. The reflexes that "open up" the circulation during vigorous exercise are not reversed quickly upon cessation of exercise. Further, when a person goes abruptly from strenuous exercise to complete inactivity, he loses a natural means of making the circulatory adjustment. That is, his muscles—which normally function as a "pump" in helping to return blood to the heart—are turned off abruptly if the exercise is ended suddenly. The circulation, then, is still opened up without the "muscle pump" to help return blood flow to the heart. With a lessened return, the heart beats more weakly, causing a rapid drop in blood pressure. In many persons, this is enough to compromise the flow to the brain—causing them to "pass out." We avoid this by making a slow and gradual transition from the vigorous exercise to the resting state. After jogging, for example, you should always walk for a period of time—usually about two to three minutes.

**Post-Workout Shower:** Since a hot shower also results in opening up the circulation, it is important that the post-workout shower be delayed until the circulatory system has returned to the normal, resting state. Depending on the weather, I would recommend waiting a minimum of five to ten minutes. Even then, the shower should be only comfortably *warm*; not hot.

**Breath-Holding:** Avoid any exercise which requires breath-holding. In any exercise which involves "straining," excessive blood pressure response will occur. As we mentioned previously, "straining" refers to the situation in which the glottis (opening between the vocal cords) is closed and pressure is built up in the chest and abdominal cavities. This type of straining is a necessary part of isometric exercise, which has become part of the vogue in recent years. Isometrics have nothing to contribute to the conditioning of older people, and should be avoided.

**Competition:** Never compete in a conditioning workout. If you work out with one or more friends, it is unlikely that the exercise responses will be alike, or even similar. Therefore, reserve your competition to vying only with yourself and then only for physical improvement as measured by the PPR and your sense of well-being! A sense of competition can be self-defeating in two ways: It might cause you to overdo in your workout, and it results in a greater flow of adrenaline. These are very undesirable effects because they make your heart action less efficient. If competition is important to you, at least restrain yourself until you achieve top-level physical fitness. And then restrict the competition to those in your own age bracket who are equally conditioned.

**Illness:** You must remember that your conditioning program constitutes a challenge to your system, a challenge which has been designed to bring about the best possible improvements in your fitness. However, if you have even a light cold, you have a second challenger. When this is added to the normal and desirable exercise, it constitutes too great a total challenge. As I have pointed out, too large a challenge is just as bad as none. Consequently, you will derive no benefits from working out when you don't feel well. In fact you will probably just slow down your conditioning progress. You might also delay the recovery from the cold or other disability. A good rule of thumb is: Don't go back to your exercise program until your energy level is back to normal. If there is any feeling of "dragging" or malaise, forget the workouts temporarily—concentrate on beating down the bug that bit you. This will require rest and following your doctor's instructions.

**In Closing:** Let me wish you success in your new physical conditioning program. I can only hope that your rewards will be as rich as those I have gained from the active life!

# CHAPTER NOTES


**Chapter 1**

1. From *Time* magazine (Feb. 7, 1969) 39. Reprinted by permission from *Time*, The Weekly Newsmagazine; Copyright Time Inc.
2. H. A. deVries, "Physiological Effects of an Exercise Training Regimen Upon Men Aged 52-88," *Journal of Gerontology*, 25 (1970), 325-336.

**Chapter 2**

1. Interview with A. E. David Schonfield, byUSC News Bureau (M. Briley) for news release dated Jan. 23, 1968.
2. H. A. deVries, "Prescription of Exercise for Older Men from Telemetered Exercise Stress Data," *Geriatrics*, 26 (1971), 102-111.
3. J. S. Skinner, J. O. Holloszy, and T. K. Cureton, "Effects of a Program of Endurance Exercises on Physical Work Capacity and Anthropometric Measurements of 15 Middle-Aged Men," *American Journal of Cardiology*, 14 (1964), 747-752.
4. H. A. deVries, "Physiological Effects of an Exercise Training Regimen Upon Men Aged 52-88," *Journal of Gerontology*, 25 (1970), 325-336.

**Chapter 3**

1. I. Zamir, "A Mathematical Model for the Prediction of Peak to Peak Torque Needed to Move the Human Middle Finger," *Ampersand Semi Annual Report*, Highland View Hospital, Cleveland, Ohio, Jan. 1966.
2. J. P. Henry and J. C. Cassel, "Psychosocial Factors in Essential Hypertension," *American Journal of Epidemiology*, 90 (1969), 171-200.
3. J. L. Boyer and F. W. Kasch, "Exercise Therapy in Hypertensive Men," *Journal of the American Medical Association*, 211 (1970), 1668-1671.
4. R. W. Eckstein, "Effect of Exercise and Coronary Artery Narrowing on Coronary Collateral Circulation," *Circulation Research*, 5 (1957), 230-235.
5. S. M. Fox and W. L. Haskell, "Physical Activity and the Prevention of Coronary Heart Disease," *Bulletin of the New York Academy of Medicine*, 44 (1968), 950-967.
6. H. A. deVries and G. M. Adams, "An EMG Comparison of Single Doses of Exercise and Meprobamate, as to Effects on Muscular Relaxation," *American Journal of Physical Medicine*, 51 (1972), 130-141.

**Chapter 4**

1. E. Hultman, "Physiological Role of Muscle Glycogen in Man with Special Reference to Exercise," American Heart Association Monograph #15 (New York: American Heart Association, 1967), pp. 99-112.
2. H. A. deVries, "Method for Evaluation of Muscle Fatigue and Endurance from Electromyographic Fatigue Curves," *American Journal of Physical Medicine*, 47 (1968), 125-135.
3. H. A. deVries, "EMG Fatigue Curves ın Postural Muscles. Possible Etiology for Idiopathic Low Back Pain," *ibid.*, 175-181.

**Chapter 5**

1. E. Jacobson, *Progressive Relaxation* (Chicago: The University of Chicago Press, 1938).
2. E. Jacobson, ed., *Tension in Medicine* (Springfield, Ill.: Charles C. Thomas, 1967).
3. H. A. deVries and G. M. Adams, "Electromyographic Comparison of Single Doses of Exercise and Meprobamate as to Effects on Muscular Relaxation," *American Journal of Physical Medicine*, 51 (1972), 130-141.
4. G. B. Haugen, H. H. Dixon, and H. A. Dickel, *A Therapy for Anxiety Tension Reactions* (New York: Macmillan, 1960).

**Chapter 6**

1. R. J. Johns and V. Wright, "Relative Importance of Various Tissues in Joint Stiffness," *Journal of Applied Physiology*, 17 (1962), 824-828.
2. W. H. Akeson *et al.*, "The Connective Tissue Response to Immobility: An Accelerated Aging Response?" *Experimental Gerontology*, 3 (1968), 289-301.
3. H. Sobel, "Some Investigations on the Role of Connective Tissue in Gerontology," in *Medical and Clinical Aspects of Aging*, ed. H. T. Blumenthal (New York: Columbia University Press, 1962).
4. N. M. Hajek, M. E. Godbey, and H. M. Hines, "Functional Changes in Muscle and Nerve Resulting from Prolonged States of Shortening," *Archives of Physical Medicine*, 28 (1947), 690-694.

5. H. A. deVries, "Quantitative Electromyographic Evaluation of the Spasm Theory for Muscle Pain," *American Journal of Physical Medicine*, 45 (1966), 119-134.
6. H. A. deVries, "Evaluation of Static Stretching Procedures for Improvement of Flexibility," *Research Quarterly*, 33 (1962), 222-229.
7. E. A. Chapman, "Effects of Exercise Upon Joint Mobility of Young and Old Men" (Unpublished doctoral dissertation, University of Southern California, 1971).

**Chapter 7**

1. F. L. Benoit, R. L. Martin, and R. H. Watten, "Changes in Body Composition During Weight Reduction in Obesity," *Annals of Internal Medicine*, 63 (1965), 604-612.
2. J. A. Greene, "A Clinical Study of the Etiology of Obesity," *Annals of Internal Medicine*, 12 (1939), 1797-1803.
3. J. Pariskova, "Impact of Age, Diet, and Exercise on Man's Body Composition," in *International Research in Sport and Physical Education*, eds. E. Jokl and E. Simon (Springfield, Ill.: Charles C. Thomas, 1964).
4. J. Mayer *et al.*, "Exercise, Food Intake, and Body Weight in Normal Rats and Genetically Obese Adult Mice," *American Journal of Physiology*, 177 (1954), 544.

**Chapter 8**

1. T. K. Cureton, "Review of Research to Determine Cardiovascular Condition (1941-1950)," in *Proceedings of the Fifty-sixth Annual Convention AAHPER* (Detroit, 1951), 167-177.
2. W. W. Waxman, "Physical Fitness Development for Adults in the YMCA," in *Exercise and Fitness* (New York: The Athletic Institute, 1960), Chap. 17.

**Chapter 9**

1. H. A. deVries, "EMG Fatigue Curves in Postural Muscles: Possible Etiology for Idiopathic Low Back Pain," *American Journal of Physical Medicine*, 47 (1968), 175-181.
2. H. A. deVries, "Electromyographic Observations of the Effects of Static Stretching Upon Muscular Distress," *Research Quarterly*, 32 (1961), 468-479.
3. H. A. deVries, "Quantitative Electromyographic Evaluation of the Spasm Theory for Muscle Pain," *American Journal of Physical Medicine*, 45 (1966), 119-134.

**Chapter 11**

1. H. A. deVries, "Prescription of Exercise for Older Men from Telemetered Exercise Stress Data," *Geriatrics*, 26 (1971), 102-111.
2. H. A. deVries, "Exercise Intensity Threshold for Improvement of Cardiovascular-Respiratory Function in Older Men," *Geriatrics*, 26 (1971), 94-101.
3. I. Astrand, A. Guharay, and J. Wahren, "Circulatory Responses to Arm Exercise with Different Arm Positions," *Journal of Applied Physiology*, 25 (1968), 528-532; U. Freyschuss and T. Strandell, "Circulatory Adaptation to One and Two Leg Exercises in Supine Position," *ibid.*, 511-515; A. R. Lind and G. W. McNicol, "Cardiovascular Responses to Holding and Carrying Weights by Hand and by Shoulder Harness," *ibid.*, 261-267.
4. A. R. Lind and G. W. McNicol, "Circulatory Responses to Sustained Hand-Grip Contractions Performed During Other Exercise both Rhythmic and Static," *Journal of Physiology*, 192 (1967), 595-607.
5. H. A. deVries and G. M. Adams, "Effect of the Type of Exercise Upon the Work of the Heart in Older Men," unpublished.
6. H. A. deVries, "Quantitative Electromyographic Evaluation of the Spasm Theory for Muscle Pain," *American Journal of Physical Medicine*, 45 (1966), 119-134.
7. H. A. deVries, "Evaluation of Static Stretching Procedures for Improvement of Flexibility," *Research Quarterly*, 33 (1962), 222-229.

## APPENDIX

### Table A

**Table for Conversion of Time for 20 Beats to Heart Rate per Minute**

| *Time* | *H.R.* | *Time* | *H.R.* | *Time* | *H.R.* | *Time* | *H.R.* |
|---|---|---|---|---|---|---|---|
| 20.0 | 60 | 16.3 | 74 | 12.6 | 95 | 9.0 | 133 |
| 19.9 | 60 | 16.2 | 74 | 12.5 | 96 | 8.9 | 135 |
| 19.8 | 61 | 16.1 | 75 | 12.4 | 97 | 8.8 | 136 |
| 19.7 | 61 | 16.0 | 75 | 12.3 | 98 | 8.7 | 138 |
| 19.6 | 61 | 15.9 | 75 | 12.2 | 98 | 8.6 | 140 |
| 19.5 | 62 | 15.8 | 76 | 12.1 | 99 | 8.5 | 141 |
| 19.4 | 62 | 15.7 | 76 | 12.0 | 100 | 8.4 | 143 |
| 19.3 | 62 | 15.6 | 77 | 11.9 | 101 | 8.3 | 145 |
| 19.2 | 63 | 15.5 | 77 | 11.8 | 102 | 8.2 | 146 |
| 19.1 | 63 | 15.4 | 78 | 11.7 | 103 | 8.1 | 148 |
| 19.0 | 63 | 15.3 | 78 | 11.6 | 103 | 8.0 | 150 |
| 18.9 | 63 | 15.2 | 79 | 11.5 | 104 | 7.9 | 152 |
| 18.8 | 64 | 15.1 | 79 | 11.4 | 105 | 7.8 | 154 |
| 18.7 | 64 | 15.0 | 80 | 11.3 | 106 | 7.7 | 156 |
| 18.6 | 65 | 14.9 | 81 | 11.2 | 107 | 7.6 | 158 |
| 18.5 | 65 | 14.8 | 81 | 11.1 | 108 | 7.5 | 160 |
| 18.4 | 65 | 14.7 | 82 | 11.0 | 109 | 7.4 | 162 |
| 18.3 | 66 | 14.6 | 82 | 10.9 | 110 | 7.3 | 164 |
| 18.2 | 66 | 14.5 | 83 | 10.8 | 111 | 7.2 | 167 |
| 18.1 | 66 | 14.4 | 83 | 10.7 | 112 | 7.1 | 169 |
| 18.0 | 67 | 14.3 | 84 | 10.6 | 113 | 7.0 | 171 |
| 17.9 | 67 | 14.2 | 85 | 10.5 | 114 | 6.9 | 174 |
| 17.8 | 67 | 14.1 | 85 | 10.4 | 115 | 6.8 | 176 |
| 17.7 | 68 | 14.0 | 86 | 10.3 | 116 | 6.7 | 179 |
| 17.6 | 68 | 13.9 | 86 | 10.2 | 117 | 6.6 | 182 |
| 17.5 | 69 | 13.8 | 87 | 10.1 | 118 | 6.5 | 185 |
| 17.4 | 69 | 13.7 | 88 | 10.0 | 120 | 6.4 | 188 |
| 17.3 | 69 | 13.6 | 88 | 9.9 | 121 | 6.3 | 190 |
| 17.2 | 70 | 13.5 | 89 | 9.8 | 122 | 6.2 | 194 |
| 17.1 | 70 | 13.4 | 89 | 9.7 | 124 | 6.1 | 197 |
| 17.0 | 71 | 13.3 | 90 | 9.6 | 125 | 6.0 | 200 |
| 16.9 | 71 | 13.2 | 91 | 9.5 | 126 | 5.9 | 203 |
| 16.8 | 71 | 13.1 | 92 | 9.4 | 128 | 5.8 | 207 |
| 16.7 | 72 | 13.0 | 92 | 9.3 | 129 | 5.7 | 211 |
| 16.6 | 72 | 12.9 | 93 | 9.2 | 130 | 5.6 | 214 |
| 16.5 | 73 | 12.8 | 94 | 9.1 | 132 | 5.5 | 218 |
| 16.4 | 73 | 12.7 | 94 | | | | |

**Table B**

**Conversion of Beats Counted in 10 Seconds to Heart Rate per Minute**

| Beats in 10 seconds | Heart rate beats/min. |
|---|---|
| 10 | 60 |
| 11 | 66 |
| 12 | 72 |
| 13 | 78 |
| 14 | 84 |
| 15 | 90 |
| 16 | 96 |
| 17 | 102 |
| 18 | 108 |
| 19 | 114 |
| 20 | 120 |
| 21 | 126 |
| 22 | 132 |
| 23 | 138 |
| 24 | 144 |
| 25 | 150 |
| 26 | 156 |
| 27 | 162 |
| 28 | 168 |
| 29 | 174 |

**Table C**

**Scoring Table for Progressive Pulse Rate Test* (Before Conditioning)**

| Classification | Total 2 minute pulse count after 12 4 step cycles per min. | after 18 4 step cycles per min. | after 24 4 step cycles per min. | after 30 4 step cycles per min. |
|---|---|---|---|---|
| | 102 | 110 | 114 | 125 |
| | 106 | 114 | 118 | 130 |
| Excellent | 110 | 118 | 122 | 135 |
| | 114 | 122 | 126 | 140 |
| | 118 | 126 | 130 | 145 |
| | 122 | 130 | 134 | 150 |
| | 126 | 134 | 138 | 155 |
| Above Average | 130 | 138 | 142 | 160 |
| | 134 | 142 | 146 | 165 |
| | 138 | 146 | 150 | 170 |
| | 142 | 150 | 154 | 175 |
| | 146 | 154 | 158 | 180 |
| Average | 150 | 158 | 162 | 185 |
| | 154 | 162 | 166 | 190 |
| | 158 | 166 | 170 | 195 |
| | 162 | 170 | 174 | 200 |
| | 166 | 174 | 178 | 205 |
| Below Average | 170 | 178 | 182 | 210 |
| | 174 | 182 | 186 | 215 |
| | 178 | 186 | 190 | 220 |
| | 182 | 190 | 194 | 225 |
| | 186 | 194 | 198 | 230 |
| Poor | 190 | 198 | 202 | 235 |
| | 194 | 202 | 206 | 240 |
| | 198 | 206 | 210 | 245 |

*H. A. deVries, K. S. Ambe, and G. M. Adams, Unpublished data.

**Table C**

**Scoring Table for Progressive Pulse Rate Test* (After 6 Weeks of Conditioning)**

| Classification | Total 2 minute pulse count: after 12 4 step cycles per min. | after 18 4 step cycles per min. | after 24 4 step cycles per min. | after 30 4 step cycles per min. |
|---|---|---|---|---|
| | 102 | 110 | 114 | 125 |
| | 106 | 114 | 118 | 130 |
| Excellent | 110 | 118 | 122 | 135 |
| | 114 | 122 | 126 | 140 |
| | 118 | 126 | 130 | 145 |
| | 122 | 130 | 134 | 150 |
| | 126 | 134 | 138 | 155 |
| Above Average | 130 | 138 | 142 | 160 |
| | 134 | 142 | 146 | 165 |
| | 138 | 146 | 150 | 170 |
| | 142 | 150 | 154 | 175 |
| | 146 | 154 | 158 | 180 |
| Average | 150 | 158 | 162 | 185 |
| | 154 | 162 | 166 | 190 |
| | 158 | 166 | 170 | 195 |
| | 162 | 170 | 174 | 200 |
| | 166 | 174 | 178 | 205 |
| Below Average | 170 | 178 | 182 | 210 |
| | 174 | 182 | 186 | 215 |
| | 178 | 186 | 190 | 220 |
| | 182 | 190 | 194 | 225 |
| | 186 | 194 | 198 | 230 |
| Poor | 190 | 198 | 202 | 235 |
| | 194 | 202 | 206 | 240 |
| | 198 | 206 | 210 | 245 |

*H.A. de Vries, K.S. Ambe, and G.M. Adams, Unpublished data.

**Table C**

**Scoring Table for Progressive Pulse Rate Test* (After 12 Weeks of Conditioning)**

| Classification | Total 2 minute pulse count | | | |
|---|---|---|---|---|
| | after 12 4 step cycles per min. | after 18 4 step cycles per min. | after 24 4 step cycles per min. | after 30 4 step cycles per min. |
| | 102 | 110 | 114 | 125 |
| | 106 | 114 | 118 | 130 |
| Excellent | 110 | 118 | 122 | 135 |
| | 114 | 122 | 126 | 140 |
| | 118 | 126 | 130 | 145 |
| | 122 | 130 | 134 | 150 |
| | 126 | 134 | 138 | 155 |
| Above Average | 130 | 138 | 142 | 160 |
| | 134 | 142 | 146 | 165 |
| | 138 | 146 | 150 | 170 |
| | 142 | 150 | 154 | 175 |
| | 146 | 154 | 158 | 180 |
| Average | 150 | 158 | 162 | 185 |
| | 154 | 162 | 166 | 190 |
| | 158 | 166 | 170 | 195 |
| | 162 | 170 | 174 | 200 |
| | 166 | 174 | 178 | 205 |
| Below Average | 170 | 178 | 182 | 210 |
| | 174 | 182 | 186 | 215 |
| | 178 | 186 | 190 | 220 |
| | 182 | 190 | 194 | 225 |
| | 186 | 194 | 198 | 230 |
| Poor | 190 | 198 | 202 | 235 |
| | 194 | 202 | 206 | 240 |
| | 198 | 206 | 210 | 245 |

*H.A. deVries, K.S. Ambe, and G.M. Adams, Unpublished data.

**Table C**

**Scoring Table for Progressive Pulse Rate Test* (After 24 Weeks of Conditioning)**

| Classification | Total 2 minute pulse count | | | |
|---|---|---|---|---|
| | after 12 4 step cycles per min. | after 18 4 step cycles per min. | after 24 4 step cycles per min. | after 30 4 step cycles per min. |
| | 102 | 110 | 114 | 125 |
| | 106 | 114 | 118 | 130 |
| Excellent | 110 | 118 | 122 | 135 |
| | 114 | 122 | 126 | 140 |
| | 118 | 126 | 130 | 145 |
| | 122 | 130 | 134 | 150 |
| | 126 | 134 | 138 | 155 |
| Above Average | 130 | 138 | 142 | 160 |
| | 134 | 142 | 146 | 165 |
| | 138 | 146 | 150 | 170 |
| | 142 | 150 | 154 | 175 |
| | 146 | 154 | 158 | 180 |
| Average | 150 | 158 | 162 | 185 |
| | 154 | 162 | 166 | 190 |
| | 158 | 166 | 170 | 195 |
| | 162 | 170 | 174 | 200 |
| | 166 | 174 | 178 | 205 |
| Below Average | 170 | 178 | 182 | 210 |
| | 174 | 182 | 186 | 215 |
| | 178 | 186 | 190 | 220 |
| | 182 | 190 | 194 | 225 |
| | 186 | 194 | 198 | 230 |
| Poor | 190 | 198 | 202 | 235 |
| | 194 | 202 | 206 | 240 |
| | 198 | 206 | 210 | 245 |

*H.A. deVries, K.S. Ambe, and G.M. Adams, Unpublished data.

**Table C**

**Scoring Table for Progressive Pulse Rate Test* (After 1 Year of Conditioning)**

| Classification | Total 2 minute pulse count | | | |
|---|---|---|---|---|
| | after 12 4 step cycles per min. | after 18 4 step cycles per min. | after 24 4 step cycles per min. | after 30 4 step cycles per min. |
| Excellent | 102 | 110 | 114 | 125 |
| | 106 | 114 | 118 | 130 |
| | 110 | 118 | 122 | 135 |
| | 114 | 122 | 126 | 140 |
| | 118 | 126 | 130 | 145 |
| Above Average | 122 | 130 | 134 | 150 |
| | 126 | 134 | 138 | 155 |
| | 130 | 138 | 142 | 160 |
| | 134 | 142 | 146 | 165 |
| | 138 | 146 | 150 | 170 |
| Average | 142 | 150 | 154 | 175 |
| | 146 | 154 | 158 | 180 |
| | 150 | 158 | 162 | 185 |
| | 154 | 162 | 166 | 190 |
| | 158 | 166 | 170 | 195 |
| Below Average | 162 | 170 | 174 | 200 |
| | 166 | 174 | 178 | 205 |
| | 170 | 178 | 182 | 210 |
| | 174 | 182 | 186 | 215 |
| | 178 | 186 | 190 | 220 |
| Poor | 182 | 190 | 194 | 225 |
| | 186 | 194 | 198 | 230 |
| | 190 | 198 | 202 | 235 |
| | 194 | 202 | 206 | 240 |
| | 198 | 206 | 210 | 245 |

*H.A. deVries, K.S. Ambe, and G.M. Adams, Unpublished data.

**Table D**

**Progress in Progressive Walking Program—Level I (First 6 Weeks)**

Name____________________________ Age_____ Resting heart rate _______________

| Exercise Progression | Date | HR | Date | HR | Date | HR | Date | HR |
|---|---|---|---|---|---|---|---|---|
| 1. Walk one mile in 20 minutes | | | | | | | | |
| 2. " 1¼ miles 25 " | | | | | | | | |
| 3. " 1½ " 30 " | | | | | | | | |
| 4. " 1¾ " 35 " | | | | | | | | |
| 5. " 2 " 40 " | | | | | | | | |
| 6. " 2¼ " 45 " | | | | | | | | |
| 7. " 2½ " 50 " | | | | | | | | |
| 8. " 2¾ " 55 " | | | | | | | | |
| 9. " 3 " 1:00 hour | | | | | | | | |
| 10. " 2 " 32 minutes | | | | | | | | |
| 11. " 2¼ " 36 " | | | | | | | | |
| 12. " 2½ " 40 " | | | | | | | | |
| 13. " 2¾ " 44 " | | | | | | | | |
| 14. " 3 " 48 " | | | | | | | | |
| 15 " 3¼ " 52 " | | | | | | | | |
| 16. " 3½ " 56 " | | | | | | | | |
| 17. " 3¾ " 1:00 hour | | | | | | | | |
| 18. " 4 " 1:04 " | | | | | | | | |

**Table D**

**Progress in Progressive Walking Program—Level I (Second 6 Weeks)**

Name________________________________ Age_____ Resting heart rate____________________

| Exercise Progression | | | | | | Date | HR | Date | HR | Date | HR | Date | HR |
|---|---|---|---|---|---|---|---|---|---|---|---|---|---|
| 1. | Walk | one | mile in | 20 | minutes | | | | | | | | |
| 2. | " | 1¼ | miles | 25 | " | | | | | | | | |
| 3. | " | 1½ | " | 30 | " | | | | | | | | |
| 4. | " | 1¾ | " | 35 | " | | | | | | | | |
| 5. | " | 2 | " | 40 | " | | | | | | | | |
| 6. | " | 2¼ | " | 45 | " | | | | | | | | |
| 7. | " | 2½ | " | 50 | " | | | | | | | | |
| 8. | " | 2¾ | " | 55 | " | | | | | | | | |
| 9. | " | 3 | " | 1:00 | hour | | | | | | | | |
| 10. | " | 2 | " | 32 | minutes | | | | | | | | |
| 11. | " | 2¼ | " | 36 | " | | | | | | | | |
| 12. | " | 2½ | " | 40 | " | | | | | | | | |
| 13. | " | 2¾ | " | 44 | " | | | | | | | | |
| 14. | " | 3 | " | 48 | " | | | | | | | | |
| 15. | " | 3¼ | " | 52 | " | | | | | | | | |
| 16. | " | 3½ | " | 56 | " | | | | | | | | |
| 17. | " | 3¾ | " | 1:00 | hour | | | | | | | | |
| 18 | " | 4 | " | 1:04 | " | | | | | | | | |

**Table E**

**Progress in Jog-Walk Program—Level II (First Six Weeks)**

Name____________________ Age______ Resting heart rate________________

| Date | | | | | | | | | | | | | | | | | | |
|---|---|---|---|---|---|---|---|---|---|---|---|---|---|---|---|---|---|---|
| 1. No. of steps in jog interval | | | | | | | | | | | | | | | | | | |
| 2. No. of steps in walk interval | | | | | | | | | | | | | | | | | | |
| 3. No. of steps of jog-walk | | | | | | | | | | | | | | | | | | |
| 4. Heart rate end of first jog | | | | | | | | | | | | | | | | | | |
| 5. " 2nd " | | | | | | | | | | | | | | | | | | |
| 6. " 3rd " | | | | | | | | | | | | | | | | | | |
| 7. " 4th " | | | | | | | | | | | | | | | | | | |
| 8. " 5th " | | | | | | | | | | | | | | | | | | |
| 9. " 6th " | | | | | | | | | | | | | | | | | | |
| 10. " 7th " | | | | | | | | | | | | | | | | | | |
| 11. " 8th " | | | | | | | | | | | | | | | | | | |
| 12. " 9th " | | | | | | | | | | | | | | | | | | |
| 13. " 10th " | | | | | | | | | | | | | | | | | | |

**Table E**

**Progress in Jog-Walk Program—Level II (Second 6 Weeks)**

Name________________________ Age_____ Resting heart rate______________

| Date | | | | | | | | | | | | | | | | | | |
|---|---|---|---|---|---|---|---|---|---|---|---|---|---|---|---|---|---|---|
| 1. No. of steps in jog interval | | | | | | | | | | | | | | | | | | |
| 2. No. of steps in walk interval | | | | | | | | | | | | | | | | | | |
| 3. No. of sets of jog-walk | | | | | | | | | | | | | | | | | | |
| 4. Heart rate end of first jog | | | | | | | | | | | | | | | | | | |
| 5. " 2nd " | | | | | | | | | | | | | | | | | | |
| 6. " 3rd " | | | | | | | | | | | | | | | | | | |
| 7. " 4th " | | | | | | | | | | | | | | | | | | |
| 8. " 5th " | | | | | | | | | | | | | | | | | | |
| 9. " 6th " | | | | | | | | | | | | | | | | | | |
| 10. " 7th " | | | | | | | | | | | | | | | | | | |
| 11. " 8th " | | | | | | | | | | | | | | | | | | |
| 12. " 9th " | | | | | | | | | | | | | | | | | | |
| 13. " 10th " | | | | | | | | | | | | | | | | | | |

**Table E**

**Progress in Jog-Walk Program — Level II (Third 6 Weeks)**

Name ______________________ Age _____ Resting heart rate ______________

| Date | | | | | | | | | | | | | | | | | | |
|---|---|---|---|---|---|---|---|---|---|---|---|---|---|---|---|---|---|---|
| 1. No. of steps in jog interval | | | | | | | | | | | | | | | | | | |
| 2. No. of steps in walk interval | | | | | | | | | | | | | | | | | | |
| 3. No. of sets of jog-walk | | | | | | | | | | | | | | | | | | |
| 4. Heart rate end of first jog | | | | | | | | | | | | | | | | | | |
| 5. " 2nd " | | | | | | | | | | | | | | | | | | |
| 6. " 3rd " | | | | | | | | | | | | | | | | | | |
| 7. " 4th " | | | | | | | | | | | | | | | | | | |
| 8. " 5th " | | | | | | | | | | | | | | | | | | |
| 9. " 6th " | | | | | | | | | | | | | | | | | | |
| 10. " 7th " | | | | | | | | | | | | | | | | | | |
| 11. " 8th " | | | | | | | | | | | | | | | | | | |
| 12. " 9th " | | | | | | | | | | | | | | | | | | |
| 13. " 10th " | | | | | | | | | | | | | | | | | | |

**Table E**

**Progress in Jog-Walk Program — Level II (Fourth 6 Weeks)**

Name ______________________ Age _____ Resting heart rate ______________________

| | | | | | | | | | | | | | | | | | | |
|---|---|---|---|---|---|---|---|---|---|---|---|---|---|---|---|---|---|---|
| Date | | | | | | | | | | | | | | | | | | |
| 1. No. of steps in jog interval | | | | | | | | | | | | | | | | | | |
| 2. No. of steps in walk interval | | | | | | | | | | | | | | | | | | |
| 3. No. of sets of jog-walk | | | | | | | | | | | | | | | | | | |
| 4. Heart rate end of first jog | | | | | | | | | | | | | | | | | | |
| 5. " 2nd " | | | | | | | | | | | | | | | | | | |
| 6. " 3rd " | | | | | | | | | | | | | | | | | | |
| 7. " 4th " | | | | | | | | | | | | | | | | | | |
| 8. " 5th " | | | | | | | | | | | | | | | | | | |
| 9. " 6th " | | | | | | | | | | | | | | | | | | |
| 10. " 7th " | | | | | | | | | | | | | | | | | | |
| 11. " 8th " | | | | | | | | | | | | | | | | | | |
| 12. " 9th " | | | | | | | | | | | | | | | | | | |
| 13. " 10th " | | | | | | | | | | | | | | | | | | |

## PERSONAL NOTES

# PERSONAL NOTES

## PERSONAL NOTES

## PERSONAL NOTES

## PERSONAL NOTES

# Index